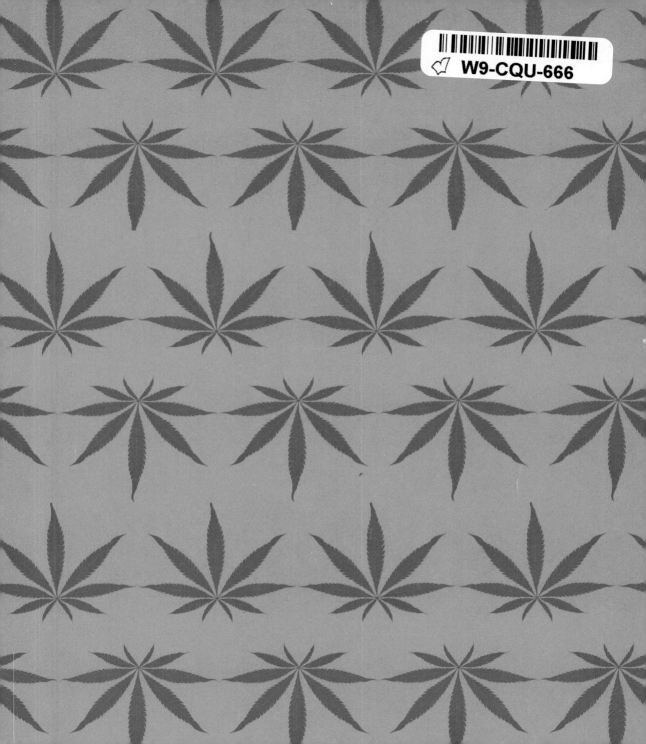

W9-CQU-666

GANJA
YOGA

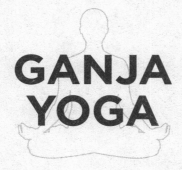

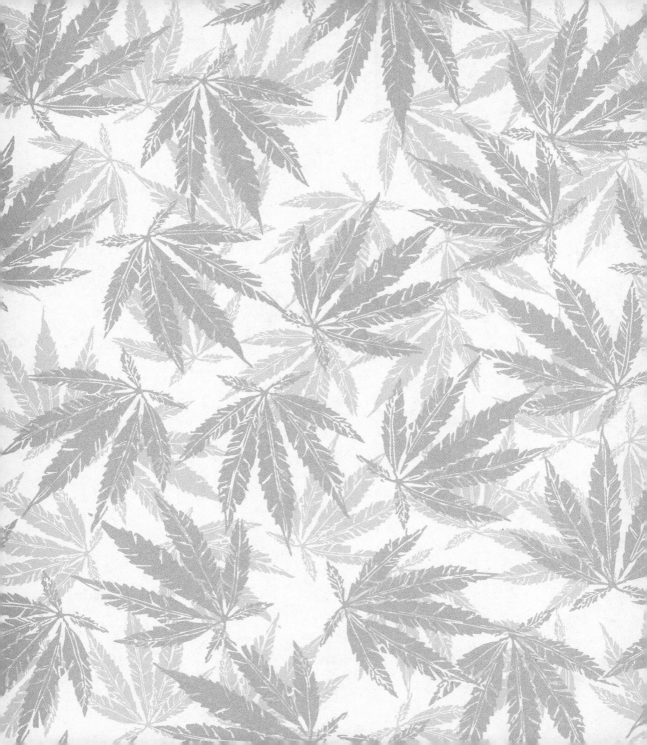

GANJA YOGA

A PRACTICAL GUIDE TO CONSCIOUS RELAXATION, SOOTHING PAIN RELIEF, AND ENLIGHTENED SELF-DISCOVERY

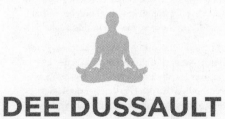

DEE DUSSAULT

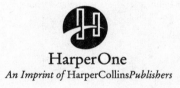

HarperOne
An Imprint of HarperCollins*Publishers*

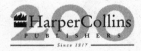

Illustrations on pages 186–187 Copyright © 2017 by Georgia Bardi.

Photographs pages 5, 20, 107, 147, and 177 by Monica Lo.

Photographs pages 154 and 270 by Anna MacKenzie.

Photograph page 50 by Gizella Olivo.

This book contains advice and information relating to health care. It is not intended to replace medical advice and should be used to supplement rather than replace regular care by your doctor. It is recommended that you seek your physician's advice before embarking on any medical program or treatment. All efforts have been made to ensure the accuracy of the information contained in this book as of the date of publication. The publisher and the author disclaim liability for any medical outcomes that may occur as a result of applying the methods suggested in this book.

GANJA YOGA. Copyright © 2017 by Dee Dussault. All rights reserved. Printed in the United States of America. No part of this book may be used or reproduced in any manner whatsoever without written permission except in the case of brief quotations embodied in critical articles and reviews. For information, address HarperCollins Publishers, 195 Broadway, New York, NY 10007.

HarperCollins books may be purchased for educational, business, or sales promotional use. For information, please email the Special Markets Department at SPsales@harpercollins.com.

FIRST EDITION

Designed by Renata De Oliveira

Library of Congress Cataloging-in-Publication Data is available upon request.

ISBN 978–0–06–265684–1

17 18 19 20 21   LSC   10 9 8 7 6 5 4 3 2 1

Dedicated to my husband,
my third love after yoga and weed.

CONTENTS

INTRODUCTION:
INVITING MARY JANE TO YOUR YOGA PRACTICE

BHAVA NA SANA HRIDAYAM.
May this cannabis be a blessing to my heart.

The first few times I consumed cannabis were so unremarkable that I can't recall them, but my third experience was a doozy. I was fifteen, in high school, adventurous, and ready for my long-promised adulthood. I can still see it: My boyfriend standing in the kitchen, his stringy black hair hanging down in his face, intently heating butter knives to red-hot on the stovetop. When they were ready, he dropped a huge plop of hash onto each of the knives, and then showed me how to sip the thick smoke through a funnel we'd fashioned from a half-gallon pop bottle.

Inhale. It doesn't feel that rebellious, really. After all, Mom smokes weed. *Hold.* Ouch, this burns. *Exhale.* Immediately the room is spinning, I can't breathe, and my heartbeat is pounding in my head. I flail about, a fish out of water, knocking over the coffee table. The room closes in around me. I'm tripping balls. *Panic attack.*

As a kid, I believed everything. *D.A.R.E.* (Drug Abuse Resistance Education) taught me about the evils of marijuana. I knew my mom did "drugs" in the back room; I could smell the skunky smoke and requisite Lysol each time and see the butts in the ashtrays after parties.

My aunt and grandmother did not do drugs, and I could tell they thought my mom should not either; their hints and indirect negative remarks were not lost on me. For my part, I was just worried about her, because I didn't want her brain to be fried like the eggs in the frying pan on TV.

One day in the sixth grade the police came to my school and showed us dirty bongs made of pop bottles, warning us about criminals who might offer them to us. I secretly died of embarrassment, certain mine was the only mother who had such paraphernalia at home. At a slumber party a year later, my friends found a baggie in my mom's bedroom. I vehemently denied it was "dope," even though they all knew it was. My plausible deniability was shattered after that, and I couldn't pretend Mom wasn't a druggie, a criminal, an outlaw. In protest, I refused to wash her dirty ashtrays.

It's no wonder, then, with visions of vicious criminals and brain cells cooking at a high temperature, that I struggled with anxiety when I did smoke. In addition to the anxiety, every time I got high after that, the intense sensation of panic would come back, a symptom of PTSD. I'd project negative meaning onto everything anyone said, or, weirder, I'd have the overwhelming sense that I could hear people's thoughts or "know" that they were reading mine. And it was always negative. I spent many nights at teenage parties bawling my eyes out, trying to just be normal and get high *like everyone else*.

After a while, I gave up trying, assuming I must have an allergy to weed. I viewed cannabis the way I did booze: a drug that is fine for my mom and friends—and even my friends who were now puffing with Mom!—but not for me.

The irony is not lost on me that I had such a negative experience with the plant early on, and now I am one of the leaders in the cannabis wellness movement. Much of my life consists of talking about how cannabis enhances my mind-body connection when I do yoga. When I think about how intense and awful that experience with weed was in my teens in light of my career, it's like talking about two different drugs.

Twelve years later when I bravely tried cannabis again, I actively strove to overcome the paranoia and dissociative states. If I microdosed, I could mitigate most of the anxiety, and getting stoned was fun. By then I had practiced a lot of yoga while sober, giving me the tools to deal with hard stuff that came up. I was older, more psychologically mature, more knowledgeable about the plant, and, not to be overlooked, not overdosing with a bunch of sweaty teenage boys.

My relationship with yoga was far less traumatic. Slow, mindful yoga had helped me through a bout of depression in my teens, had given solace to my feelings of isolation and loneliness at college, and had soothed my nerves as I went through breakups in my twenties. I even brought it with me when I taught English in South Korea for two years. It's my longest-lasting friendship.

So when I developed a healthy relationship with weed—finally— the first thing I noticed is that it made yoga, like sex and music, *far better*.

I could quiet my mind in ways I had never before been able to do, despite my many years on the mat. Pot lifted a veil of mental fog that I didn't even know existed. It's a little like the years I'd spent thinking my digestion issues were normal, until a friend (correctly) suggested maybe I was lactose intolerant. When I cut out dairy, my bloating disappeared and my definition of "normal" totally changed.

With the addition of ganja, my definition of "yoga" would never be the same. I could get to bliss and clarity in my meditations far faster and deeper than when sober. The mental chatter slowed down, and I could more easily connect with the profound space and silence inside.

Plus, I could finally *feel* the esoteric aspects of yoga that I'd been reading about for years, things like *chakras*, which in yoga are seven "vortexes of energy" that run along the spine and have a coordinating color and psychological association. Being a smarty-pants, I've always valued the rational mind and didn't believe in anything that couldn't be proven by science. Meditating on my heart, throat, or third eye when doing yoga sober rarely felt any different from focusing on the palm of my hand, lip, or any other nonchakra part. After I enhanced yoga with cannabis, however, the subtle yet not-so-subtle pulse of aliveness in these "energy centers" could not be denied, despite my rational academic mind's disbelief in them.

Not only did I feel chakras when I did stoned yoga, I found myself experiencing orgasmic bliss from them! Spirals of cascading pleasure and delight with no beginning and no end. Yum!

Needless to say, these fruitful experiments propelled me to start blending cannabis and yoga practice regularly. This was before major news outlets were publishing front-page stories about the medical benefits of weed. It was also before I knew yogis in India had been elevating the practice for millennia. I just know it worked for me, which is surprising because I was twenty-seven and had been doing yoga since I was fifteen. As I said, I was a late bloomer.

Despite still having to grapple with paranoia at times, I found that pot brought unmistakable insight to my life and yoga practice. I learned to work *with* my cannabis-fueled anxiety, realizing that the plant had been magnifying some of the thoughts and feelings I had not been allowing myself to express, negative emotional stuff that had been bottled up for years, even decades.

Weed-fueled yoga made the high feel psychologically and spiritually therapeutic, like the way peyote and ayahuasca might work. Journeys into some of the darker parts of the self can sometimes be painful, but with my twelve-year yoga practice now enhanced with cannabis, I could tap into and heal things I hadn't before been able to access. *While doing yoga.*

I also loved how pot helped me tune into my body and connect to the stretching muscles. It wasn't all shamanic voyaging into darkness. In fact, it was mostly just awesome stoner trippin' and feeling groovy.

A year later, I went from fighting paranoia most of the time I got high to less than half the time. I'm a lot of things, and tenacious is one of them.

As I mastered dose and setting and brought light to my unconscious fears so they had less power, I soon started toking more often, one to three times a week. It was still very tentative. I did so only in situations where I could feel safe, be warm enough, have water handy, and be around people I was fully comfortable with. My pasties (mouth dryness), my munchies, my sense of time shifting, all the stoner stereotypes were superstrong for me then, and I was very protective of my high, especially knowing how awful it was when it slid into a bad trip.

As I got more into the ganja, I switched gears professionally. I went from working on a graduate degree in human sexuality to a five-hundred-hour yoga teacher training program. The training program was the most relaxing, "spiritual" one I could find, and it felt right for me. Later I found out it was based on Tantra Yoga and emphasized the mystical aspects of the tradition.

I developed a close relationship with my teacher, Ananda Shakti, a white woman who wears colorful Indian saris and a bindu, or ornamental dot, at her third eye (located in the middle of the forehead). Midway through the training I asked her her opinion about combining cannabis and spiritual practice.

She said sometimes regular pot use can "open unhealthy energy channels," but otherwise we each make our own path to finding oneness with all. She herself practiced without enhancements or sacraments and didn't even consume wine with dinner. But because she was not demanding that I live her life or treat her as a guru to be emulated, I got her indirect blessing for my enhanced yoga leanings, promising to keep her concern about the "additional energy channels" (which I only felt when high on pot anyway) most certainly in mind.

· · ·

I CAN'T BE SURE, but according to Google I was the first Westerner to offer yoga classes where people enhance. Ganja Yoga started as a monthly class in Toronto in 2009 in my living room. Today, eight years later, I teach two popular weekly classes and have a thriving private practice in San Francisco, where I (stereotypically?) moved.

I've taught a variety of people, including a movie star, and in a variety of different places, including on the beach in Costa Rica and at Burning Man. Other teachers in Juneau, Denver, Seattle, Honolulu, LA, and Vancouver have been inspired to offer their own version of enhanced yoga. Ganja Yoga has been covered in the *New York Times* and in news outlets from Europe to India. One day, one of the biggest and most respected publishers in the world knocked on my door (okay, sent me an e-mail). And now we have the book you hold in your hands.

I could have never foreseen what Ganja Yoga has become. It has exploded from its humble beginnings in my living room to a worldwide phenomenon, rising alongside and as a result of daily news reports on the health benefits of cannabis and the lightning-fast move toward legalization. It's a breathtaking, trippy fairy tale.

Look at me, Mom. Pretty good for a poor girl from rural Ontario.

If you have picked up this book, it means you're a part of my fairy tale now, and if I have done my job, I'll be a part of yours.

Some of you will be new to either yoga or cannabis or both. No matter where you're coming from, my philosophy is that Ganja Yoga be an expression of the accepting, easygoing attitudes stemming from both yoga and weed. Even if you're a newbie, it's all good, man.

In these pages you'll find everything you need to know for safe, relaxing experiences with weed, yoga, and the two combined. If you're already a cannabis user, whether a seasoned daily stoner or occasional toker, I hope you'll be inspired to try yoga, and especially stoned yoga. If you already practice yoga, I'd love to inspire you to try a slower, easier, more mindful practice than what's usually thought of as "yoga" and to introduce you to the wellness benefits of the complex and miraculous plant that is cannabis!

As the pioneer of this movement, I want to emphasize that Ganja Yoga is yoga for all bodies; it is able to work to some degree for anyone. If you're not sure you can do it, know that I've taught it to an eighty-year-old MS patient in a wheelchair, a man recovering from a ten-year coma, veterans, several abundant-bodied folks, and many inflexible people who claimed they couldn't "do yoga."

Cannabis-enhanced yoga (and really all yoga) is not about accomplishing poses; it is about feeling our bodies and becoming more relaxed and present. People who have felt excluded from the challenging world of modern yoga appreciate this, as do fit, healthy people who are looking for a more mindful, meditative practice than what is offered in most mainstream studios.

Ready to learn more? Let's start by diving into all the incredible things that cannabis can do for our bodies and minds. Then we'll explore the science behind the benefits of yoga before bringing the two together, which is where the magic *really* begins.

If you're already a toker, go ahead and spark up if you'd like. Weed makes yoga better, so I'm sure it also makes reading about yoga better! And if you're not sure if weed's for you, no pressure here (that wouldn't be very yogic!). We'll get to the enhancing later; I for one know that good things come to those who wait.

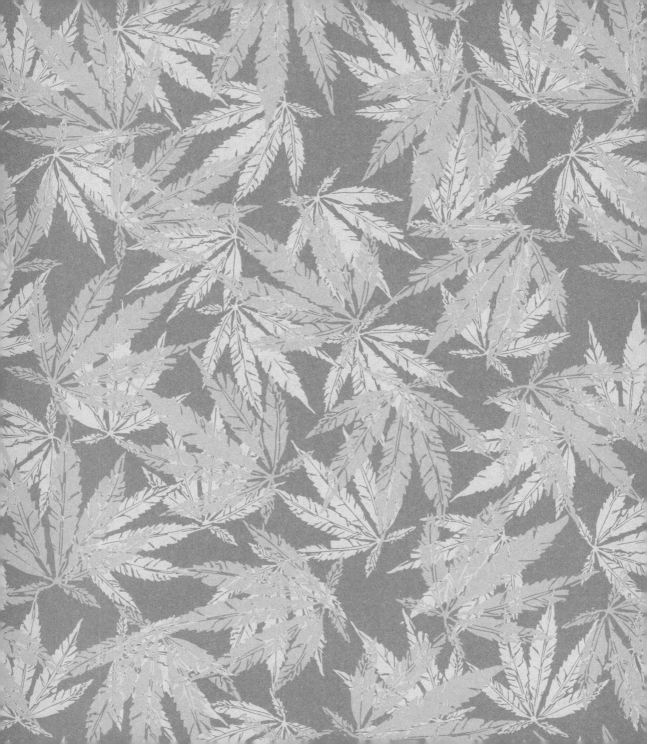

GANJA
YOGA

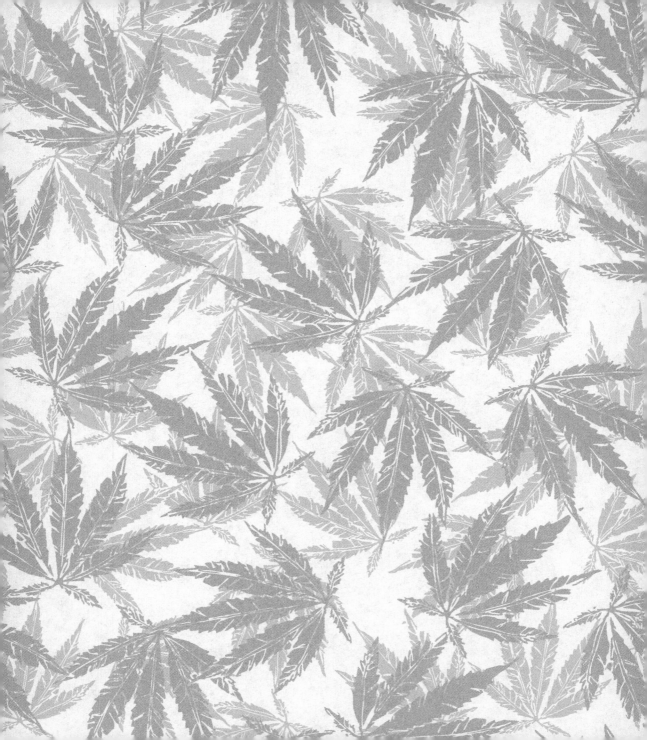

CANNABIS AS MEDICINE

GATHER ROUND, FRIENDS. I'm here to tell you about the miraculous and scientifically proven benefits of pot. If you've never smoked marijuana, this will clear up any concerns you may have about using it in a mindful way, as a healthy habit. On the other hand, if you're a longtime smoker or at least a frequent flier, this chapter will give you factual information about the natural enjoyment you already experience.

Before we begin Cannabis 101, though, it's important to note: *there's no such thing as "recreational" use.* Considering the imbalanced, incredibly stressful world we live in, all cannabis use is "medicinal." We know chronic stress is a leading cause of disease and premature death, so anything that cures or relieves the pathological tension of our times is a healer and an aid.

It isn't just a treatment, however. Cannabis is *preventive medicine,* an approach to wellness that our culture doesn't prioritize as a fundamental part of health care. In our culture we focus more on treatment than prevention. However, maintaining healthy endocannabinoid system tone, in the way we hit the gym to maintain healthy muscle tone, improves our resilience to stress and its related ailments. (The *endocannabinoid system,* ECS, is a signaling system in the brain that produces natural endocannabinoids to help regulate body processes such as appetite, pain, mood, and memory, in much the same way that the brain uses other neurotransmitters such as dopamine and serotonin to regulate other systems.)

Regular doses of cannabis, rather than larger amounts less frequently, are a tonic to support a powerful healing system for mental health and wellness.

Whether we have a natural deficiency or a stressful and imbalanced lifestyle, cannabis can be a dietary supplement much like other supplements we take: vitamins, minerals, amino acids, or omega-3 fatty acids. It can be put under the tongue in a flavorless tincture, added to any type of food, rubbed onto aching muscles, vaped (the vapor inhaled) discreetly and easily, or smoked the good old-fashioned way. It can get you outer-space high, make you slightly intoxicated, or not affect you mentally at all.

Cannabis should not be seen as a form of "complementary" or "alternative" medicine. Cannabis is a nutritional supplement that millions of people all over the world already use to cope with the stresses of modern living. More and more sensible people are turning to it for this reason, as well as for its anticarcinogenic, antioxidant, anti-inflammatory, anti-anxiety and antidepressive, neuroprotectant, and pain-killing properties.

Cannabis is the most widely used medicinal substance in the world. It's been used this way for thousands of years. It's one of humanity's oldest cultivated crops. With education and some trial and error, each person can form a unique relationship to this herbal remedy to treat and prevent countless common ailments!

The Benefits of Bud

Highly versatile, cannabis safely provides relief from many different ailments and symptoms, as shown by scientific studies. The National Organization for the Reform of Marijuana Laws states: "Despite the US government's nearly century-long prohibition of the plant, cannabis is nonetheless one of the most investigated therapeutically active substances in history." Some of the many conditions that cannabis, in one form or another, has been unequivocally shown to treat include:

Pain	**Nausea**
Inflammation	**Glaucoma**
Anxiety	**Migraines**
Depression	**ADHD**
Seizures (in conditions like epilepsy)	**PTSD**

It also helps people with AIDS manage their symptoms and may also slow down the progression of the disease. It has been shown to slow the growth and spread of cancer under laboratory conditions.

Contrary to the message of those sizzling eggs that so terrified me long ago, cannabis is actually a neuroprotectant, which means it safeguards the brain's cells from oxidation and other forms of damage and degeneration, which is helpful for patients suffering from disorders like Alzheimer's and Parkinson's disease. Some research suggests cannabis may even be a preventative for these diseases.

Weed also improves blood-sugar levels, helpful for anyone but especially for those with diabetes. People who medicate with it regularly also have healthier body mass indexes, smaller waist sizes, faster metabolisms, and higher levels of good cholesterol!

The enormous benefits are unmistakable. **Cannabis is medicine.** Although research on cannabis and health is still in its infancy, the implications are enormous and can remove the stigma surrounding the plant once and for all.

Now we're going to learn more about the components that make up the plant, focusing on the two most popular cannabinoids: cannabidiol (CBD) and tetrahydrocannabinol (THC).

CBD: The Wonder Drug

Although THC is far more well known, I want to start with CBD, for it truly is a miracle worker and is only recently getting the attention it deserves.

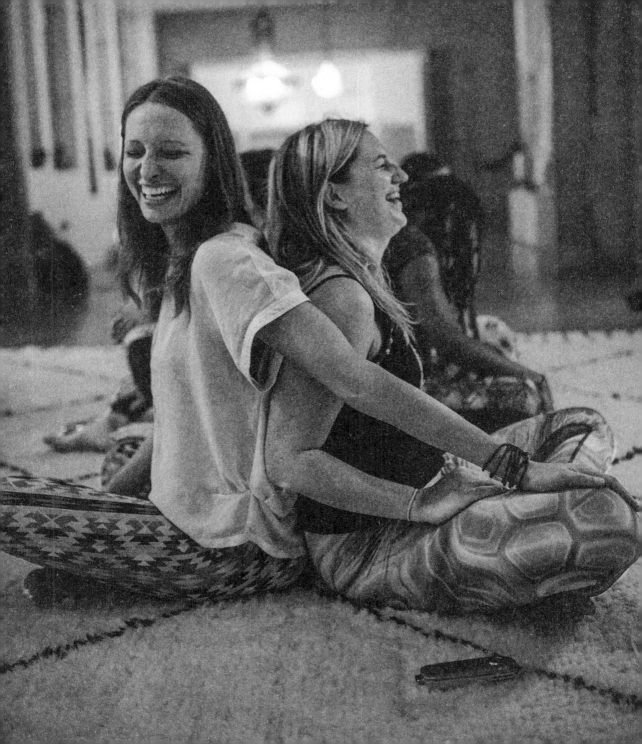

CBD IS SAFE

A recent review of the available literature on CBD found: "Several studies suggest that CBD is non-toxic in non-transformed cells and does not induce changes in food intake, does not induce catalepsy, does not affect physiological parameters (heart rate, blood pressure, and body temperature), does not affect gastrointestinal transit, and does not alter psychomotor or psychological functions. Also, chronic use and high doses up to 1,500 milligrams a day of CBD are reportedly well tolerated in humans." The same review reported comparatively minor side effects: drug interactions (via the same compound that makes grapefruit interact with some drugs), sleepiness, and, most seriously, *potential* impacts on fertility and in vitro cell viability.

A DETERRENT TO OPIOID OVERDOSE

Every day over forty Americans die from accidentally overdosing on prescription painkillers. Many of these people were using a drug they were prescribed (and, tragically, many of the prescriptions were addictive opioids that, had cannabis been available, would not have been needed in the first place). In less than twenty years, deaths from prescription opioid overdose have *quadrupled*; prescription opiates now kill more people than suicide and motor-vehicle deaths combined. The situation is now considered an "epidemic" by the Centers for Disease Control and Prevention. CBD can be used to prevent addiction (and resulting accidental overdose) to pharmaceutical opioids. In states where cannabis has been legalized, deaths from prescription painkillers have gone down 25 percent and addiction to them has declined markedly. However, this is only the beginning of the immense healing ability of one of humanity's most beneficial herbs.

HEALTH BENEFITS

What I find most exciting is the fact that CBD has been demonstrated to be a highly effective analgesic (treatment for generalized or acute pain). I watched my mom struggle with crippling fibromyalgia and arthritis (in one study, CBD actually blocked the progression of a type of arthritis); if **pain relief** was all CBD did for health, it would be enough for me to sing its praises.

When an injury occurs, white blood cells fill the injury site as a protective measure. This is one cause of inflammation. The other cause is stress. When no injury is present, inflammation starts in the gut lining, which can cause ailments in other body parts or stay in the gut as an inflammatory bowel disorder such as Crohn's disease, irritable bowel syndrome, or celiac disease.

Inflammation is an immune response that's been implicated in many conditions, like diabetes, heart disease, migraines, dental issues, obesity, cancer, and pain. CBD has been shown to have strong **anti-inflammatory** qualities, providing those white blood cells with a little rest and relaxation.

In this fast-paced, ultrabusy, downright f'd-up world of ours, depression and anxiety run rampant. So many of us have anxiety-induced digestive disorders and sleep disorders, not to mention substance abuse

Studies have failed to show any brain damage from cannabis. A recent study on rhesus monkeys used technology so sensitive that scientists could actually see the effect of learning on brain cells, and it found cannabis caused no damage.

or struggles with suicidal thoughts related to the stress and sadness in our lives. CBD has **anti-anxiety** properties; it has been shown to elevate mood while also reducing symptoms of generalized anxiety, panic attacks, and post-traumatic stress disorder (PTSD).

Along with its painkilling, anti-anxiety, and anti-inflammatory properties, CBD is an **antioxidant,** which means it prevents cell damage and aging.

It's the CBD in cannabis that blocks deposits in the brain that cause **Alzheimer's**. It's also been shown to dramatically reduce muscle spasms and seizures in people suffering from a **spasmodic disorder.** Finally, CBD is a promising treatment for **heart health,** reducing oxidative stress and fibrosis in heart cells.

And, with regard to CBD's **cancer-fighting** ability, it is *cytotoxic,* which means it turns off a gene that expresses and spreads cancer! In both test tubes and animal studies, CBD has shown a remarkable ability to stop the proliferation of cancer cells. This finding has exciting implications for thousands of people. While we wait for more research to verify this effect and to find the appropriate dosing amounts, CBD is also already helping to reduce chemo-induced neuropathy and nausea in cancer patients.

(NOT) TRIPPIN'

CBD is not psychoactive. Although it fosters a sense of well-being, it doesn't cause the reality-altering feeling of being "high." This is good news for the huge number of people who are wary of cannabis because of the psychoactive experience; they can now receive the health benefits as well! Many states have legalized agricultural production of industrial hemp, from which CBD can be obtained for therapeutic use.

The cool thing is, many people who try CBD for the first time, myself included, feel as though a veil has been lifted. We become aware of the low-level anxiety and constant mental contraction we endure in our day-to-day lives. It's hard to explain, but with CBD something shifts. The world seems lighter, friendlier. Whether this is indeed a mild psychoactive effect or something else, I'm not sure, but it's mind-blowing (without being mind-bending).

Considering these incredible health benefits, it isn't hard to see how CBD can be of benefit to *everyone*. Now let's learn more about THC, the poster child for pot as we typically think of it.

THC: The Health Tonic That Gets You High

THC is the most commonly occurring and well known compound in cannabis, for it is the one that leads to psychoactive highs. It is the stuff that makes conversations free and fun, comedy even more hilarious, sex even more orgasmic, and chocolate mousse even more . . .

Where was I?

THC is indeed the most abundant cannabinoid in most strains of weed available today. For this reason, THC has mistakenly been called the "active ingredient." This is a misconception.

When the other cannabinoids are selectively bred out of cannabis so there is more THC and the "high" is stronger (which is what most cultivators have done until recently), we unwittingly lose many of the positive effects of the herb, while opening ourselves up to the potential for increased anxiety, the very thing we already have too much of in our world.

Because of something called the "entourage effect" CBD (and other cannabinoids) must be present in cannabis to counter the potential adverse effects of THC. The entourage effect essentially says that the compounds in cannabis work better together than in isolation. Because we have been obsessed with THC for so long, we are only *now* learning the value of the other, equally "active" cannabinoids. However, even modern pharmaceutical companies like GW Pharmaceuticals, maker of Sativex for multiple sclerosis patients, have embraced whole-plant medicine.

THC has many therapeutic properties. Like CBD, THC is anti-inflammatory (twenty times more powerful than aspirin and twice the amount of hydrocortisone). And like CBD, it has antinauseant, neuro-protective, and antioxidant properties. In petri studies, THC stops the spread of brain cancer. It's also a bronchodilator, easing breathing for those with respiratory ailments like asthma.

CBD and THC: The Next Generation

Until recently, because THC was known to be the main psychoactive component of cannabis, cultivators concentrated on it. In an illicit market stronger is always better, so it wasn't worth getting to know the other cannabinoids. Nowadays, CBD and the other eighty or so cannabinoids

SLOW SCIENCE

If there's anything we know from science, it's how much we don't know.

For example, did you know there's a nerve in the brain that was only discovered recently? It had to be named "zero" because nerves one through twelve had already been taught in medical schools for decades. Its existence may suggest humans also use pheromones to attract a mate, as other animals do.

Did you know there's a web of connective tissue called fascia that surrounds the muscles, nerves, and organs, yet most medical textbooks make little mention of it? Anatomical representations always show the tissues stripped of the fascia, because we cut the cadavers in medical school the way we butcher our meat.

And of course there's the crucial cannabinoid system, which regulates a number of other systems in the body but was only discovered in 1990!

are all being recognized as an exciting part of cannabis wellness, especially for people interested in exploring the benefits of cannabis without the anxiety that THC can sometimes bring.

Ganja certainly has profound health effects on the human body. Now on to yoga.

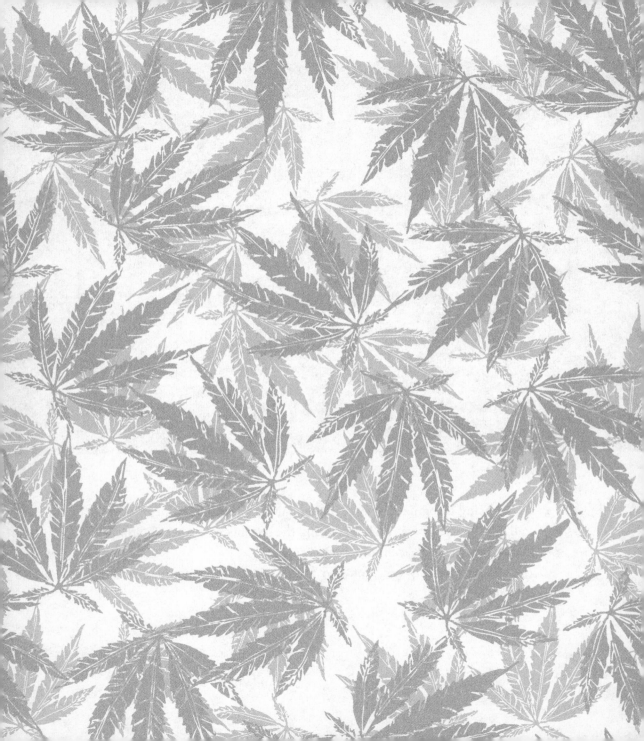

WHAT YOGA CAN DO FOR YOU

REGARDLESS OF WHETHER you've never done a Downward Dog in your life or your day is not complete without a little time on the mat, you're probably aware of the many health benefits the practice of yoga offers. That said, you may not know *all* of the reasons why yoga rules. There are too many to count here, but here's my personal list of the top ten most compelling reasons why you should get your yoga on, stoned or not.

1. Yoga makes positive physiological changes in the brain.

Meditation and movement have both been proven to be successful treatments for depression, anxiety, and other mood disorders. In a recent study, the combination of thirty minutes of meditation and thirty minutes of moderate aerobic exercise twice a week brought reduced brain activity linked to negative rumination, and the depressed reported a 40 percent reduction in their symptoms. Researchers suggested the permanent brain changes may be linked to a reduction in stress hormones or the fact that movement creates more of the biochemicals in the brain that are responsible for improved mental health.

Practicing yoga increases gamma-aminobutyric acid (GABA), a neurotransmitter in the brain that regulates neurons by keeping them from overfiring and overwhelming the nervous system. People with depression or anxiety tend to have lower levels of GABA, the body's natural Valium, so a little yoga can (literally) give them a boost. Yoga also thickens the layers of the cerebral cortex, the part of the brain associated with higher cognitive functioning. This increases *neuroplasticity,* which is the scientific word for new brain grooves. These new grooves are what help us learn new things and break unhealthy habits.

2. Stretching relaxes the nervous system.

By activating the parasympathetic part of the body's nervous system, the heart rate, blood pressure, and breathing all slow down, which brings profound physical and psychological stress-relieving benefits. Numerous scientific studies have shown the importance of a daily relaxation practice to treat and prevent a vast array of conditions, including hypertension, arthritis, insomnia, depression, infertility, cancer, anxiety, and even aging. Although there are many ways to relax our hyperaroused nervous systems, like soaking in a warm bath, walking in nature, or hot sex, yoga calms the nervous system while at the same time slowly coaxing shortened muscles back to their proper length. Parasympathetic nervous system activation (e.g., bending your body like a noodle) leads to daydreaming, thinking, and reflection, a different state of consciousness than we experience in our busy daily lives. As well, recent animal studies have shown stretching to be anti-inflammatory, and we all know how important that is!

3. Movement improves circulation of nutrients throughout the body.

Short muscles and stiff joints mean decreased blood flow and resulting cellular degeneration. You may not know this, but exercise only brings circulation to the body parts that are being used in the movement, not to the whole body. Most modern workout programs leave many parts of the body undermoved, reducing circulation of nutrients into the tissues. Yoga, with its varied postures and movements, is one of the healthiest ways to truly stay fit, helping the muscles, organs, glands, tissues, and systems move nutrients in and filter waste out.

RUNNER'S HIGH

Endorphins are the body's natural opioids, similar to many prescription painkillers and heroin. They're often given the credit for the feeling of euphoria that comes after a workout. However, new research has shown it is not endorphins but in fact endocannabinoids, your body's natural cannabinoids, that cause "runner's high" after exercising. Both are released into the bloodstream, but scientists have shown that endocannabinoids are what's responsible for the relaxation that comes after a really good yoga session.

4. Movement now keeps us moving later.

Movement patterns we establish now will give us increased ability to move well later in life. We are a sedentary culture. When we don't move, as when we sit for ten hours a day most days, we get "adhesions" on the body's connective tissues. These inelastic pieces of scar tissue hinder mobility, causing pain, and result in overcompensation and injury in the surrounding tissues. Movement will keep the muscles long, the joints flexible, and the whole body supple and limber. There is an ego boost to being able to touch your toes, but health into old age is the real benefit of flexibility!

5. Relaxation restores the adrenal glands, and they need it badly.

The American Psychological Association reports that 75 percent of Americans report suffering from high or moderate levels of stress. Our adrenal glands help us to deal with stress by releasing cortisol, a hormone that helps the body respond to stressful situations. However, if we are under constant stress, even at a low level, it is theorized that our adrenals become triggered by increasingly smaller stressors and start to flood the body with cortisol and adrenaline more and more often. The constant background hum of the triggering of the "fight or flight" response is the cause of most of our agitation, tension, anxiety, and unhappiness. When high levels of stress hormones are secreted often, they can even lead to stress-related medical conditions like cardiovascular disease, gastrointestinal diseases, sleep disorders, weight gain, and memory and concentration impairment. Relaxation-based yoga restores the damage caused by overuse of the adrenal glands.

6. Relaxation releases emotional tension.

Emotional tension can be shaken off during yoga movements, and unconsciously held stress can be released from the psyche without even needing to look at the contents. Many yoga practices include letting out big yawns and sighs to exorcise mental and emotional tension with sound vibration. And it definitely costs less than your therapy appointment.

7. Yoga can help us to be less reactive.

In the yogic space of awareness, all feelings, sensations, thoughts, and impressions are allowed to arise. The practice is to notice and release whatever comes up. Over time, this mindful practice decreases the power our emotions have over us, since we can watch them as they arise without giving in to the habit of reacting to them. As well, our nervous systems become more regulated and less reactive to stress. In time, yoga practitioners begin to live more harmoniously with themselves and others.

8. It's just good to be quiet sometimes.

Quietness is rarely encouraged in our culture. Whether in our free time or at work, attaining more material accomplishments is considered more important than developing a connection with one's body, emotions, creative self, or intuition. Yoga says that by focusing only on outward paths to happiness we strengthen the ego, which is the limited sense of separate self we all have to some degree. In the long run, these superficial pursuits only leave us more tense and anxious, more separate and fearful; the way we chase happiness in fact causing us more pain. Yoga practitioners across time and place have all said that in taking time to get quiet and connect within, we are able to tap into an infinite source of inner peace and connection with others. Moments of quietness are extremely restorative and are painfully lacking in our day-to-day lives.

9. Yoga is easy and enjoyable!

Yoga is safe, affordable, easy to learn, suitable for all bodies, and, most important, fun! It offers many opportunities for creativity and play and lots of diversity in movement types to ensure your joints get rotated in all positions and all your muscles get strengthened, lengthened, and massaged.

10. Yoga can be transformative— I'm living proof!

Most people go through life completely unaware of how much inner tension they carry. Even when they're sleeping, tensions and worries swirl around in their heads, so they wake up just as tired, once more facing a whole new day to go through on autopilot, a day in which the constant mental noise will once again drain their energy reserves.

As we practice mindfulness and yoga, we start to become aware of the insane internal tensions we all carry, which is the first step to letting them go. Releasing tension frees up energy in unimaginable ways.

When I started to develop my sense of awareness in meditation, I was really angry at myself for tolerating so much ongoing mental garbage for so long. Then I realized I was beating myself up, which was just more inner tension! My teacher assured us that it's normal to be shocked at what's inside as we start the mindful practice of yoga, but that over time these basic mental tensions will all be released: the judgments of others, the self-hatred, the habits and rigidity of thought that limit us, and the "stickiness" of it all. As we view them dispassionately and accept them,

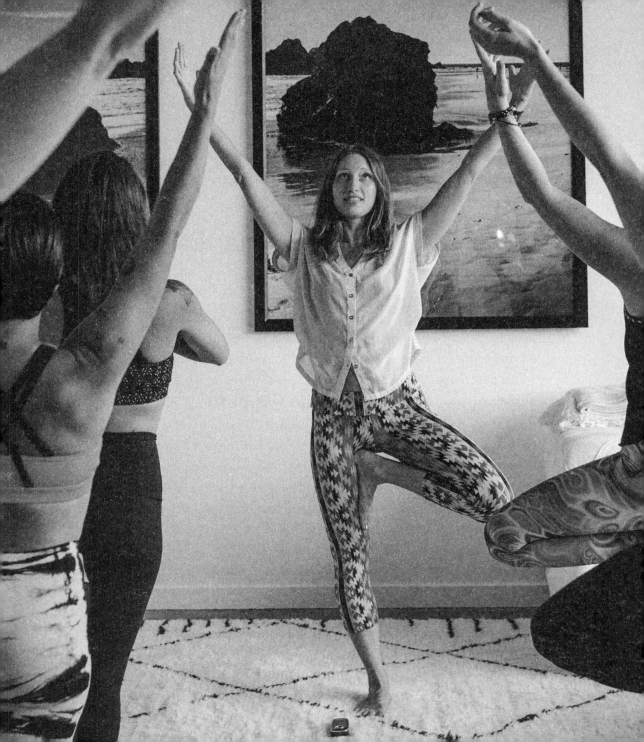

Mindfulness, breathing, movements, and meditations form a complete yoga practice that will certainly leave you more relaxed and positive. If you also find you become more awake to the reality of your true nature, which is a lot less limited than you think, that's wonderful. If you come to be a lot more appreciative of the exquisite beauty that exists around you, also great. But if not, even relaxation is a "spiritual" transformation in times as crazy as ours!

Self-care is a priority, not a luxury.

we can truly give them all away and release ourselves from their power to control us. This shit works.

After releasing surface tensions, yoga practitioners are able to access some of the deeper parts of the mind, an expansion of consciousness that many people never experience, a connection to deeper aspects of self, beyond tension and noise.

All yoga, as vast and varied as the practices are, has one thing in common: to bring a sense of meaning and joy to the practitioner's life, a chance to explore the recesses of the mind, and to eventually realize one's true nature, which is connection to all things. As we see these deeper parts of ourselves, we transform in ways that may be hard to imagine from the outset. Yoga definitely can change a life that feels stuck or unfulfilling. Habits of being, thinking, and acting get shifted when we become more self-aware. It's an applied science, a way of engineering "heaven on earth."

However, in case you're worried, yoga doesn't require you to ascribe to the philosophy of yoga! Yoga is a spiritual practice, but it also considers itself a science in which *you* are the experimenter *and* laboratory. You do the practices, then decide for yourself if your quality of life is improved. That's all. You don't have to change your beliefs or lifestyle.

You don't have to become "spiritual"—you just have to do yoga.

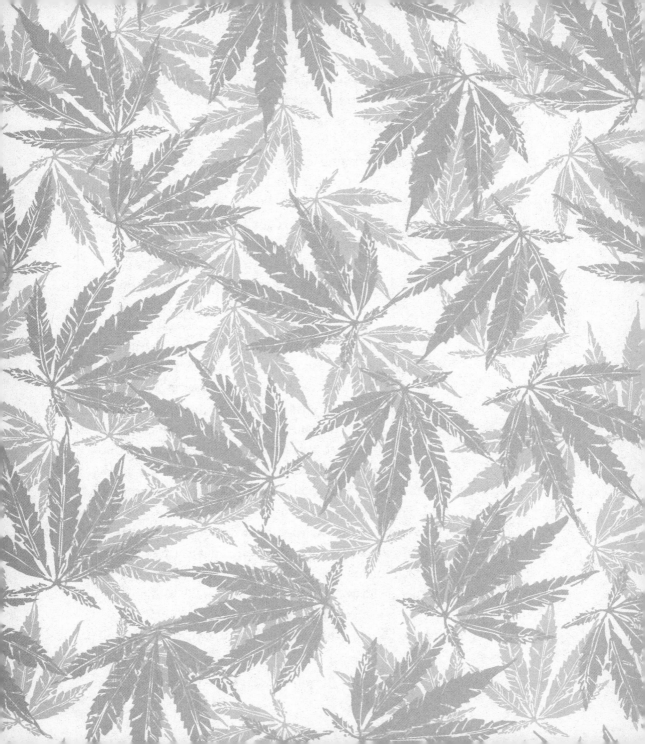

3

YOGA AND CANNABIS:
Spirituality's Virtuous Cycle

IT'S CLEAR THAT BOTH YOGA and cannabis offer a ridiculous number of health benefits, even for people who aren't drawn to the spiritual aspects.

For those that *do* wish to go beyond the pragmatic applications, yoga and weed are both very effective tools for spiritual growth, or the journey toward enlightenment. They both bring a shift in consciousness that allows one to become more open to psychological, emotional, and energy states that aren't usually operational in the grind of daily life. I'll use the word "spiritual" to describe these states and feelings, but they require no specific belief system and they are open to agnostics, atheists, and any religious believers or nonbelievers.

In our culture, there is little emphasis on spiritual discovery, consciousness expansion, working with the unconscious mind, or enlightenment. These are all seen as "woo-woo" pursuits. Plus, there's no time for them when we're all working so hard and are busier than ever. We have notifications keeping us glued to our phones, news stories keeping our adrenaline pumping, millions of dollars of advertising ensuring we aren't satisfied by what we already have; we sit hours and hours in the same positions, in our cars and at our computers, making our bodies stiff and sluggish.

On top of that, all sorts of unconscious stressors drain our energy: unhealthy food, traffic, fluorescent lights, air pollution, noise pollution, and artificial environments with no access to natural landscapes. Our mass use of caffeine and alcohol does not help: both have been proven to make our stress responses worse. Simply existing in the modern world presents mental, physical, and emotional afflictions. From global threats like climate change, health epidemics, terrorism, and inequality to local issues of racism, sexism, police brutality, and destructive influences of technology, we deal with more stressors on a daily basis than people have at any other time in human history. It's no wonder a lot of us are freaking out on the inside right now, dealing with things that didn't *exist* even one generation ago.

We don't know what to do about all this negativity. We're overwhelmed, we lack guidance, and it hurts to feel, so for the most part we go to work and act normal even though our hearts are breaking. Under these circumstances, it's absolutely no wonder "spirituality" seems impossible, laughable, meaningless, or weird.

Because there's no room for spirituality in our culture, the consciousness-enhancing aspects of both cannabis and yoga are under-emphasized. Our subjective, interior experiences with these things are not valued as much as our "yoga abs" or the big bong on our coffee table. The visual cortex of the human brain is hyperdeveloped, so it makes sense to some degree, but the explanation doesn't justify the losses we suffer when we all approach life like this.

After all, our consciousness is truly what shapes our reality. The mood we're in and the framework through which we see the world impact how we relate to people and then, quite naturally, how people relate to us.

Our "ordinary states" of consciousness don't seem to be working for us very well, as evident by our numerous mental and physical imbalances. Whatever our own unique spiritual philosophy, we as a culture are exhausted, depressed, irritated, moody, and anxious. We're suffering from obesity, diabetes, heart disease, ulcers, and other stress-related illnesses at alarming rates. We need a shift.

Perhaps you already reach for a joint to step outside the noise from time to time, or you drop into a yoga class when you've had a particularly stressful week. But if you haven't combined the two, you're in for a treat. Think about it like peanut butter and chocolate: each is fantastic on its own, but when they come together, each makes the other better.

Ganja plus yoga might already make perfect sense to you. For many people, simply saying the phrase "Ganja Yoga" turns on a lightbulb, eliciting an immediate "Of course!" Regardless of your stance, the phenomenon deserves deeper exploration for deeper appreciation.

Benefits of Ganja Yoga

In spite of the fact that we all have different spiritual beliefs and goals, here are the five ways cannabis and yoga work together to help even the most cynical skeptics find sacred reprieve from the onslaught of modernity.

ENHANCED RELAXATION

According to both science and yoga, relaxation is the key to well-being. Certainly you've noticed you have more energy and feel happier when you're relaxed, whether you're hiking in nature, lying on the beach, having dinner with friends, or daydreaming on the couch. Slowing down and taking some time at that pace of life feels good.

As with all animals, relaxation is the natural state of being for humans, the one that feels the healthiest and most pleasurable. Yet as good as it feels to relax, many people find it hard to do on their own. As a species we've become so out of balance that we carry around enormous amounts of physical and mental stress and barely even register it. Creatures of habit, we're so used to living with tension that *letting it go* takes practice.

A lot of activity goes on in our prefrontal cortex—the part of our brain that is responsible for analyzing and processing information. We have very busy minds and very sedentary bodies, and it's depleting as hell. Cannabis and yoga work similarly to facilitate relaxation by activating parts of the brain other than those accessed by "ordinary waking consciousness." This brings greater introspection, daydreaming, self-examination, creativity, and play—the qualities of consciousness we enjoy when we're relaxed. And because cannabis can bring anxiety relief and muscle relaxation, it deepens the relaxation effect of yoga; the two

> "I do not consider myself a religious person in the usual senses, but there is a religious aspect to some [cannabis] highs. The heightened sensitivity in all areas gives me a feeling of communion with my surroundings, both animate and inanimate. Sometimes a kind of existential perception of the absurd comes over me and I see with awful certainty the hypocrisies and posturing of myself and my fellow men. And at other times, there is a different sense of the absurd, a playful and whimsical awareness. Cannabis brings us an awareness that we spend a lifetime being trained to overlook and forget and put out of our minds." —Carl Sagan

work symbiotically to neutralize the corrosive effect of tension.

We may feel as though we don't have the time, skills, or even permission to fully release our anxieties. The good news is that any work to cultivate relaxation is always worth the effort. Nearly everyone who gets into yoga finds that even a little consistent practice in developing relaxation brings enormous rewards later on, off the mat.

Cultivating conscious relaxation helps to deal with the stressful aspects of life in a way that is unparalleled. Mindfulness practice can be done anytime to override emotional reactivity. Meditation tends to bring relaxation of deep-seated tensions. Yoga poses relax and balance the body. Cannabis helps relax and balance the mind.

On a personal level, cannabis helps me to disengage my brain from my task lists and concerns, so I can more easily release the thoughts that distract me from my practice of mindfulness, movement, breathing, and meditation, all of which relax me further.

The main benefit of Ganja Yoga is that it helps people to tap into the relaxation response, the drive that we all have to live simpler, happier lives. That's a form of spirituality we can all get on board with.

DEEPER EMBODIMENT

Like relaxation, embodiment is another state of being that we are not culturally encouraged to cultivate. Watching TV, being on our devices, multitasking, and being preoccupied with the past or future all take us away from a connection to our body. Being *embodied* in this context means being fully aware of and present in the body, feeling connected to it when walking, jogging, doing yoga, having sex, standing in line, and even working at the computer. It's a practice, and it's also the state of being that results from the practice.

The full expression of embodiment comes naturally to all other animals, and to human children, who are very in touch with their bodily wants for touch, movement, pleasure, and novelty. It's been suggested that our deeply entrenched cultural habit of adult estrangement from our bodies is actually a form of trauma, unnatural even though widely accepted as normal.

Movement practices tend to bring the awareness into the body, so walking, sex, working out, martial arts, dancing, and of course yoga are all good places to start embodiment practice. Sensuality and sensory experiences also enhance our bodily awareness, especially luxurious fabrics and massages. Many cannabis strains also foster greater embodiment (more on that later). Students who practice yoga regularly often remark with surprise how much more deeply they can feel their bodies the first time they try cannabis-enhanced yoga. Ten years of feeling your body in a posture and then feeling your body in that posture when you're in a more open, expansive, and connected state of bodily awareness ... well, it's a totally different thing.

Because of its focus on sensation and embodiment over visual form, Ganja Yoga tends to be a more internalized experience than what many are used to from yoga. Cannabis draws the practitioner more deeply into *feeling,* so there's less mental activity related to what the teacher is saying, how to do the pose "right," or what the person on the next mat is able to do.

Movements and transitions are slow, so we can tap in and *feel.* Very soon, comparisons, "shoulds," judgments, and other distractions melt away, as we become fascinated by the aliveness inside. We learn to feel the body without judging what we feel, and over time we start to let the body dictate the poses we take and how long we hold them for, based on the intelligence we've connected to, not instructions from a teacher or video.

Embodiment is very different from the relationship we usually have with our bodies. Usually, we only notice our body if it bothers us. Cannabis-enhanced embodiment not only gets you out of your head; it brings a whole new sense of connection to yourself. The weed makes you want to lie back and feel, and then the yoga teaches you to feel in ways that others have been doing for thousands of years.

Until a singularity occurs and human beings are truly connected to machines, I urge you to remember that we are more monkey than computer. Regardless of how embodied we are or aren't, each of us is an animal, with a responsive, deeply wise body that is eager to be listened to.

Feeling a greater sense of embodiment can be truly scary when you have chronic pain. It's understandable to be tempted to do everything you can to *avoid* being in touch with the body. "Distract me with thoughts—anything—just don't make me feel." I get it.

However, when we are in conversation with the body, we can react to its messages faster, and the pain signals don't have to be as loud to get our attention. We start to take better and better care of our body, because we hear what it needs. We begin finding appreciation for how our body gets us around and brings us pleasure. We begin to view the body not as a burden, but as a sacred vehicle and best buddy, regardless of pain, extra weight, lack of flexibility, age, size, or shape.

DOUBLE YOUR PLEASURE, DOUBLE YOUR FUN

Anyone who has had stoned sex, eaten delicious food while high, or listened to favorite music while medicated knows cannabis deepens the sensory experience. In yoga practice, cannabis heightens all five senses, especially the tactile and kinesthetic sense of touch and body awareness.

At times this can mean we become even more aware of the pain and tension we're carrying. But once we notice just how awful it feels to carry it, we are truly able to let it go. When we stay blind to the tension and pain we hold in the body, we unconsciously adapt to it, and it eventually develops into more serious issues. Finally letting go of pain and tension is so pleasurable that at times my private clients actually weep from the release!

When cannabis is added, the effect is even more pronounced. I've used cannabis to journey *into* my chronic back pain, making a yoga practice of really feeling and releasing tiny muscular or energetic holds in ways that I cannot do when I don't have the added sensitivity that cannabis brings.

Most of us have no idea the amount of pleasure the body can experience. Once pain is absent or significantly reduced, we get to spend our yoga practice trancing out to the sensation of breathing or the fascinating feelings in the heart, stomach, and pelvis, yummy sensations that are always in our bodies, waiting to be noticed. I bet you didn't know pleasure was a spiritual pursuit!

Once I started incorporating cannabis into my yoga practice, I immediately tapped into increased awareness of the subtle sensations inside of myself, the more mystical aspects of yoga that aren't often talked about in America. I don't even know if I *believe* in chakras from a rational, intellectual standpoint, but when I'm elevated, I completely *feel them,* such that I even experience (hands-free) orgasmic pleasure from them!

Cannabis brings enormous insight, healing, and pleasure to what is usually a form of fitness. You've never taken a class at the gym that was as purely enjoyable as this.

ELEVATED CREATIVITY

Contrary to stoner stereotypes, cannabis has positive mental effects, particularly with regard to creativity. Studies have shown that when people are high, they make creative associations that can lead to radically new ideas. I often get incredible bursts of insight when I do yoga high, innovative perspectives on challenges that I've been rolling over in my brain and epiphanies from my little green muse.

As well as helping me to innovatively solve problems, the enhanced creativity I get from weed allows me to create new versions of standard poses, modifications to flows, and novel dance explorations that have kept my yoga practice fresh for years. Cannabis doesn't *hinder* linear thinking; it *encourages* nonlinear thinking, something most of us need to develop.

EXPANDED CONSCIOUSNESS

In tribal cultures that perform trance dances, people move their bodies to the rhythm of the drums and achieve very altered states. Sufi whirling dervishes go around and around in circles to reach an altered, or spiritual, state. Expanded consciousness can also be accessed by fasting from food for a period of time, from prolonged arousal, as in tantric sex, or via psychedelic substances like LSD, cacti, fungi, and ganja.

The word "psychedelic" means "that which reveals the mind." A *psychedelic* is a substance or experience that produces a temporary alteration in the state of consciousness, so cognition and perception are altered. The effect is temporary, but the insights gained can be permanent.

For thousands of years, yogis, mystics, and shamans from every continent around the world have been using cannabis and other plant medicines to leave behind ordinary states of consciousness and explore portals to other dimensions of experience.

Altered states range in intensity from very negative experiences on one end of the spectrum to very positive ones on the other. At the positive end are the four experiences we just discussed: relaxation, embodiment, pleasure, and creativity. Although not "mystical" per say, these are already alternatives to the consciousness that dominates our modern world, where competition and conflict are the norm.

It's truly backward that the brain waves and biochemistry associated with daydreaming, enjoying music, doodling, and feeling your body relax in the bathtub are not valued parts of our human experience! Wouldn't it be great if we lived in a culture where the frenzied multitasking mind was the "altered" state?!

Until we flip the system, "altered states" are defined as mental and emotional experiences of reality that are vastly different from what most of us have in our day-to-day lives. As we move up the spectrum of intensity, these trippy experiences become harder to explain. Time slows down, intuition is enhanced, insight flows unexpectedly, dots get connected, and life is full of meaning. When people are able to relax enough to enter alternate states, their fear-based egotistical identifications and attachments are more easily dropped. They become less concerned with material success and the opinions of other people. As a result, they feel far happier.

Altered states are a means of breaking through the barrier of our cultural conditioning into the expansive, free, information-rich universe of direct experience and infinite possibilities. They connect us to our truest selves and lead us toward our highest potential. Altering one's state of consciousness is a spiritual practice that brings healing and deeply meaningful experiences.

You haven't heard much about altered states, because they can't be co-opted by capitalism. At least not yet. Turning on and tuning in is a personal experience. At the same time, subjective altered states share many characteristics across time and place. When altered, thinking is nonlinear, and experience feels more like a poem than a narrative. This is the

It isn't just about ordinary versus nonordinary states of consciousness or stoned versus sober. Life offers us a spectrum of expanded states, even though we've been conditioned to think of things as black or white. Many people who use cannabis regularly find that their "ordinary" way of being becomes more expanded even when they aren't under the influence. Their personalities move along the spectrum, slowly but surely, to a state in which agitation and competition eventually do become "nonordinary."

realm of magic, synchronicity, and imagination, beyond words and concepts.

Deep meditation, a long period of silence, sex that seems to go on forever, an extraordinary run in nature—we've all experienced a mental or emotional state that felt "nonordinary," even if the word "spiritual" was not used. Just because we don't see these experiences and states favorably represented in the media doesn't mean they aren't amazing. They can't be sold to us, but they're cool. Just because we have trouble talking about them doesn't mean they lack real meaning.

The urge to explore nonordinary states of consciousness is a primal one, universal across continents and time, thought by many to be integral to the development of our highest selves. Some forms of Tantra Yoga consider altered states to be a pivotal step in attaining enlightenment.

Entheogens are substances that produce expanded states of consciousness for spiritual purposes. Most are illegal, like psychedelic cacti, MDMA, LSD, and magic mushrooms; some legal entheogens include cacao, kava, wine, and, depending on where you live, cannabis.

Invite altered states, expanded awareness, and mystical experiences as you do yoga and get high, and especially as you do the two together. Even if others dismiss your experiences, even if you don't understand them with your intellect, just breathe and surrender. Let yourself feel good and release control of your mind as you go deeper and deeper into the hard-to-understand-with-the-brain parts of existing. Sometimes we want our cognitive mind to be running the show, and sometimes we don't. The enriching benefits of altered states make any fears of appearing or becoming "woo-woo" seem quite silly after the fact, but believe me, I've been there. The first few times I tried ecstatic breathing, shamanic journey work, or even the altered state of cannabis, I was really afraid to go too deep. Now I love having peak experiences, incredible expanded states that are among the most meaningful in my life. Everyone starts somewhere.

Altered States, Permanent Traits

You can reach an altered state of consciousness by becoming entranced by a fire, dancing without care for a long time, spending quiet time in nature, or doing certain types of breathing exercises. You can also combine two things that already change our state of consciousness by practicing Ganja Yoga.

In any case, the more we make time to alter our state of consciousness, whether through the skillful use of cannabis, visiting the higher plane of the yoga zone, combining the two, or doing something else entirely, the bigger a part of our reality the newly expanded awareness becomes. Anything we do repeatedly creates a neural groove in the brain, so experiencing the "spiritual" aspects of life today predisposes the brain and makes it more natural in the future. In this way, cannabis use is about far, far more than the momentary high, and yoga practice goes way beyond the time on the mat.

It's important to get off the production/consumption wheel, but we sometimes need to go beyond merely relaxing. Altered states can help us to loosen the idea we have of ourselves as separate, disconnected beings (ego identification), help us shed culturally conditioned ways of being that don't serve us, and guide our sweet spirits home to enlightenment.

Your next step is to consciously "ground," or integrate, your nonordinary experiences into your everyday life. Instead of making the distinction between "how awesome you feel at Ganja Yoga" and "how much

WHAT IS ENLIGHTENMENT?

Enlightenment is something I only know intellectually. Of course I've had glimpses of it in Ganja Yoga, states of bliss that have become more frequent and longer lasting, but I am not yet residing in a continuous state of consciousness that is beyond conflict, anger, jealousy, and anxiety (especially when I'm hungry!). I'm still a child at times, full of ego. I'm definitely becoming a better human through yoga, I'm passionate about it, and I'm a good teacher, but, to be clear, I'm not an enlightened guru.

Having said that, enlightenment is the one and only goal of traditional yoga, so it's good to have an idea of what it means before we decide if it's worth pursuing. Enlightenment generally means a state in which our consciousness or awareness has evolved to the point that it remains above our culturally conditioned limitations or narcissistic self-concerns. Once we've attained enlightenment, all thoughts, words, and deeds issue from a place of union with all aspects of our self and all other beings.

Experiences can be enlightening, and we can feel more enlightened after having an experience, but we have attained a permanently enlightened state only when we feel as connected to and concerned for other beings as we do to and for ourselves. The objective is not to transcend the world or human affairs, but to be liberated from suffering and to help all humans become liberated, because we view them as extensions of ourselves, all while being completely engaged in the world.

The pursuit of enlightenment is not about pretending to be anything other than what we are. We can do good deeds and think good thoughts as a spiritual practice, but we can't force enlightenment. It's about the journey. You can't rush or fake it. The pursuit of enlightenment is not about nirvana or heaven as an "after you die" goal (although good karma results in a more auspicious birth the next time around as well). Enlightenment allows us to embrace our current incarnation, our present human experience, fully and completely. As we become more and more awake and enlightened, we feel as though we're part of an evolving universe, as if our spiritual awakening is a tiny part of the unfolding of creation itself. Needless to say, the urge to act carelessly, selfishly, and fearfully motivates us less as we experience ourselves as part of the evolutionary unfolding of life!

We're already a part of this unfolding, but we're not *aware* of it, so we're not actively participating in it. We're not conscious of the bigger context in which our life is occurring. When we awaken to that and recognize we can not only free ourselves from narcissism and ignorance, but simultaneously become one with the very force of creation, our enlightenment journey has begun. Our individual consciousness evolves, and, as we inspire others, we take part in the evolution of culture.

Enlightenment doesn't care how you get there.

Enlightenment comes from persistent practice.

you hate your regular life at your job," your yogic objective is to blend the elements to find pleasure or acceptance in *each moment*. It's a conceptual tool to call some experiences "spiritual" and the others "mundane"; the objective is to have enough of the former and bring them into the latter, so every moment becomes an opportunity for euphoric enlightenment. In Ganja Yoga, the emphasis is not on one particular static state of consciousness, but on the dynamic process of integrating the various states.

With things so busy, so imbalanced, so stressful, what I'm saying can seem like a low priority, far too much work. I get it. I'm very busy myself, and actually pretty lazy. I know it can be hard to find the time or even the desire to get off social media and do this. Plus, you probably don't have many people you trust telling you the benefits of this spirituality business, so without a model or guidebook that feels as though it speaks to you, it can be easy to mock, ignore, or give up too quickly on your enlightenment journey.

You only have to do what you want to do.

Cannabis helps to bypass conditioned mental habits like rumination and anxiety. A few minutes of mindfulness and a couple of tokes are all you need to soar directly to the more rarified and meaningful aspects of life for a while. Cannabis and yoga have been used by yogis for thousands of years precisely for this purpose, bringing them incredible serenity, sensitivity, and insight. With repeated practice, the neural groove in our brain will help us become more and more like the "best self" we experience ourselves to be while in the altered state.

For most of us, a single enhanced yoga class does not lead to permanent enlightenment. Cannabis is an accelerant to our spiritual practice, not a substitution for it. However, we have our whole lifetime (and, according to yoga, several of them), so with time and practice we can use cannabis to slowly (though not as slowly as when sober) become enlightened and evolve out of the confines of the ego, which causes us suffering. Start with what feels right to you, and if the spiritual stuff yoga offers is far too woo-woo, it truly doesn't matter. What matters is that yoga and cannabis together can create permanent positive changes to your brain and outlook on life, even after the altered state is gone.

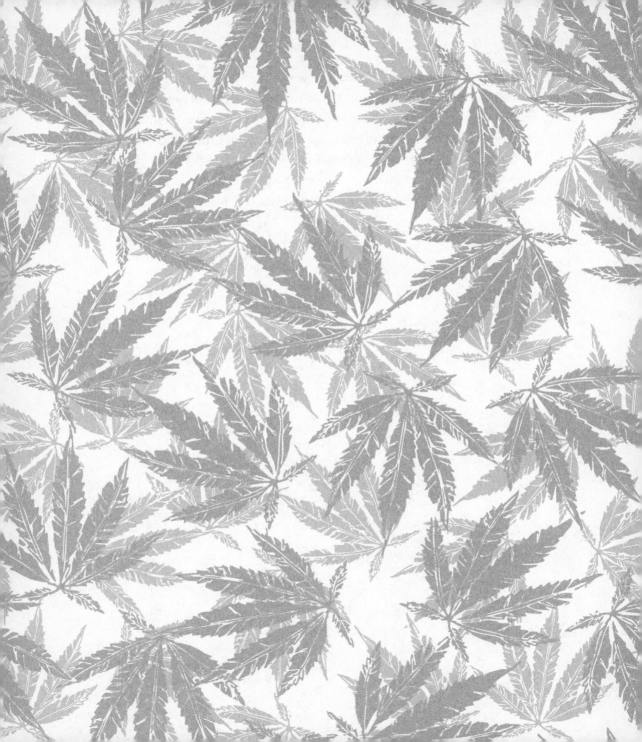

4

THE HISTORY OF CANNABIS AND YOGA

"We beseech, kindle the perfect ambrosia: the supreme nectar of sacred knowledge, the sacramental substance, here for all the assembled yogis."

—THE MAHAKALA TANTRA

SOME SPIRITUAL PRACTITIONERS question the positive impact cannabis has for spiritual practice and quality of life. For the most part, this is because they are not in possession of the facts about the plant or aware of the historical relationship between cannabis and yoga.

41

This may be a surprise, but most of the poses that we do in our modern yoga classes are less than 150 years old. Many have their roots in gymnastics, not ancient spiritual practice. What we call "yoga" is very different from what yogis were doing on the banks of the Ganges River three thousand years ago.

Yoga practitioners can find this hard to believe. We want yoga to be timeless and clean-cut: one tradition or lineage we can trace and follow, a pillar of authority we can rely on unquestioningly, or at least a few lineages and philosophies, but not a tangled web.

Truth is, the system and practice of yoga have been evolving alongside humanity since its creation. Several different waves of settlers came through the Indus Valley region of ancient India, and from the beginning the system of yoga has been a cross-stitched quilt of the various beliefs and practices of different cultures—from the Aryan Scythians to the orgiastic Kali worshippers, from the warring Sikhs to the peaceful Buddhists, with thousands of other colorful deities and experiences woven in.

The Yogic Use of Herbs

One of the more ancient aspects of yoga is the use of plant medicines. In the seminal *Yoga Sutras* (ca. 400 CE), used as a main text in most modern yoga teacher training, the path and practices for attaining enlightenment are explained by the sage Patanjali.

As elucidated in his text, five paths can be followed to gain realization of one's divine nature, the end goal of yoga. These are sheer luck (a rare occasion; for people carrying good karma from a past life), the repetition of mantras (sacred sounds), meditation practices, austerities (ascetic rituals and purification practices), and the use of certain herbs:

> *Siddhis [spiritual powers or abilities] are born of practices*
> *performed in previous births, or by herbs, mantra repetition,*
> *asceticism, or by samadhi [the end result of meditation].*
>
> SUTRA 4.1

Although it is not entirely clear which herbs he meant (because the *Yoga Sutras* are both aphoristic and metaphorical), most historians agree that Patanjali was referring to a psychoactive plant, probably cannabis, potentially mixed with other things. The *Encyclopedia Britannica* explains, "Allusions to twigs and branches suggest . . . perhaps hemp."

The guru of my yoga lineage (though not my personal guru), Swami Satyananda Saraswati (1923–2009), did not think the holy herb was cannabis. He argued that Patanjali wouldn't advocate for cannabis because, according to him, cannabis causes disease and nervous disorders. Although Satyananda's impressive list of books on yoga and his development of Yoga Nidra ("yogic sleep," or deep relaxation) are both astounding additions to the canon of yoga, being a human of the modern age, he was as affected by global antimarijuana propaganda as the rest of the world, and as a result he was totally (and understandably) dead wrong about the harms and benefits of the plant.

Far before the time of Patanjali, Satyananda, or any other teacher or guru you can name, Hinduism's most ancient scriptures (2000–1550 BCE) make direct and favorable mention of cannabis. These four books, called the Vedas, are believed by Indians to be transmissions given directly to early meditators, not created from the human mind like other books.

Veda means "to know." The oldest book of the four, the *Rig Veda,* talks about attaining spiritual states of union through cannabis, which was called *soma.* Translated from Sanskrit, a passage reads: "We have drunk *soma* and become immortal; we have attained the light, the gods [have been] discovered." The last of the holy books, the *Atharva Veda,* refers to cannabis as one of the five most sacred herbs humanity has to release anxiety; it is a "sacred grass" and a "heavenly guide."

It should be noted that some scholars do not think the elixir *soma* actually was cannabis. Unlike those in China, Siberia, and Russia, ancient burial sites in India have no archaeological evidence of cannabis. This may be because the ancient Aryans burned their dead instead of burying them, so cannabis seeds would have been destroyed. To me it's clear *soma* was cannabis. Much like the Catholic Eucharist, *soma* was prepared and consumed in a sacred ritual. It was said to bestow spiritual inspiration and good health, exactly the two benefits we know cannabis provides.

If anybody gives you heck about your weed-enhanced yoga practice, tell them the Vedas are some of the *oldest sacred texts in the world,* and they speak *openly and reverently* about (what was very probably) cannabis. **As a spiritual sacrament.**

Shiva Worship

Many people know the Indian deity Shiva is associated with yoga and cannabis. Exactly why is less known. Indian mythological tales can be quite long, so to give a brief version, our story starts when the demons and deities decided to churn the primeval ocean, what was called the "ocean of milk," because both groups wanted the prized *amrita,* the sacred nec-

"Intoxicating cannabis drink is consumed in order to liberate oneself, and those who do so, in dominating their mental faculties and following the law of Shiva [yoga], are to be likened to immortals on earth."
—*The Mahanirvana Tantra*

tar of immortality, that was said to be produced from the churning. No one group could do it on their own, so they had to work together. For the churning rope they used the hundred-headed serpent Vasuki, and for the churning pole they used Mt. Mandara. They wound the serpent around the mountain and, pulling it this way and that, splashed and dashed the ocean to and fro.

Bad news though, the churning unleashed more than just *amrita*. Up from the depths came a terrible poison, strong enough to kill all of creation. Bravely, Lord Shiva swallowed it and saved everyone. Later, when the churning finally produced *amrita* and drops of it hit the ground, cannabis sprung up, and the ever generous Shiva brought it down from Mt. Mandara for the pleasure of humankind.

Thousands of years before Patanjali's *Yoga Sutras*, Aryan priests in India would grind cannabis buds and leaves in a mortar with a pestle and mix them into clarified butter and cow's milk with fragrant spices to form a consecrated beverage that was later called *bhang*. To this day, Indian sages drink the sacred elixir for religious rites on holy days. It is used as a sacrament to Shiva, who is, surprise, surprise, the Lord of Ganja *and* the Lord of Yoga. Shiva cults are one of the oldest traditions in India.

Want to make your own ganja milkshake? Check out Appendix II.

Ayurveda, the Indian medical system that coevolved with the spiritual system of yoga, has recognized cannabis as a medicine since ancient times, using it to treat dozens of diseases and medical problems like headaches, menstrual pains, and poor appetite.

THE ORIGINAL REEFER MADNESS!

Dating to the second century BCE through the third century CE, but containing much older traditions, the Laws of Manu is an ancient legal code of Hinduism, covering norms for domestic, social, and religious life. Strongly influenced by Buddhist beliefs and practices that advocated for purity, the Laws of Manu have been interpreted to prohibit spiritual cannabis use, resulting in the tendency to criminalize its use in later centuries in India (although it should be noted that India has always been much more tolerant of cannabis than modern America).

Under the influence of global prohibition and propaganda, none of the dominant branches of yoga in America or India endorse the use of cannabis for practice, but you can still see many wandering yogis near the River Ganges and throughout India smoking their hash, drinking their ganja milkshakes, and performing *pujas* (devotions) to Lord Shiva.

Humanity Evolved with Cannabis

Sea squirts are marine organisms that shared a common ancestor with vertebrates (animals, reptiles, birds, fish, etc.) 55 million years ago. These primitive animals have a precursor to the human heart. And they have an endocannabinoid system, producing naturally occurring cannabinoids like other animals. According to NORML, "By comparing the genetics of cannabinoid receptors in different species, scientists estimate that the endocannabinoid system evolved in primitive animals over 600 million years ago."

Mind-altering plant and fungal medicines grow in every habitable place on earth. Chimps eat over a dozen species of plants for medicinal purposes. Large groups of them have been known to walk long distances to get to these medicinal plants, which scientists later discovered do things like kill parasites, fungi, and viruses. In fact, whole classes of compounds for human use have been formulated as a direct result of watching our wild cousins. Evidence from all over the world shows animals in the wild using psychoactive plants and mushrooms.

Early humans would naturally observe and learn from the animals around them, and, being animals themselves, would also be drawn to various forms of plant medicine. Modern anthropologists studying hunter-gatherer tribes found that they have an encyclopedic knowledge of local flora and fauna. The fungi, plants, and animals that they formed a special connection with were integrated into primitive spiritual rituals, rituals that would later evolve into yoga, for example.

Cannabis is known to be one of humanity's earliest agricultural crops, having evolved between 6 and 34 million years ago. The exact time and place of first contact is still debated: some scientists point toward central Asia and others identify Europe during the last Ice Age. The herb entered the archaeological record of Asia and eastern Europe at about the same time, between about 12,500 and 10,000 years ago. A recent review of cannabis archaeological data links an intensification of cannabis use in East Asia with the rise of transcontinental trade at the dawn of the Bronze Age, about 5,000 years ago.

Humans used both nonpsychoactive hemp and the more medicinal cannabis version of the plant for a variety of reasons. Perhaps it was first used for food, as it was for other animals, then as medicine, and later as an intoxicant to enter an altered state as part of spiritual rituals. At some point we began making rope and textiles from its fiber, and those ropes may have been instrumental in the domestication of the horse.

Charred seeds have been found inside the burial mounds dating back to 3,000 BCE, and the oldest cannabis archaeological relic in existence is a piece of hemp cloth from 10,000 years ago.

A fourteen-year-old girl who died giving birth in the fourth century CE was found with hash in her abdomen, likely evidence of the use of cannabis for speeding childbirth, for which it was used well into the nineteenth century.

Psychoactive plants and fungi have been used in spiritual rituals for at least eight thousand years. When civilizations began to spring up at the end of the Neolithic period, psychotropics were there. The Chinese were toking some twenty-seven hundred years ago; and the Scythians spread both cannabis and horseback warfare throughout the Eurasian landmass in the thousand years before the Common Era.

GETTING HIGH THE SCYTHIAN WAY!

Herodotus, the West's first historian, writing in the fifth century BCE, reports on the customs of the Scythians, who occupied lands northeast of the Black Sea:

> *After the burial, those engaged in it have to purify themselves, which they do in the following way. First they wet soap and wash their heads; then, in order to cleanse their bodies, they act as follows: they make a booth by fixing in the ground three sticks inclined toward one another, and stretching around them woollen felts, which they arrange so as to fit as close as possible: inside the booth a dish is placed upon the ground, into which they put a number of red-hot stones, and then add some hemp-seed.*
>
> *The Scythians, as I said, take some of this hemp-seed, and, creeping under the felt coverings, throw it upon the red-hot stones; immediately it smokes, and gives out such a vapour as no Grecian vapour-bath can exceed; the Scyths, delighted, shout for joy, and this vapour serves them instead of a waterbath; for they never by any chance wash their bodies with water.*

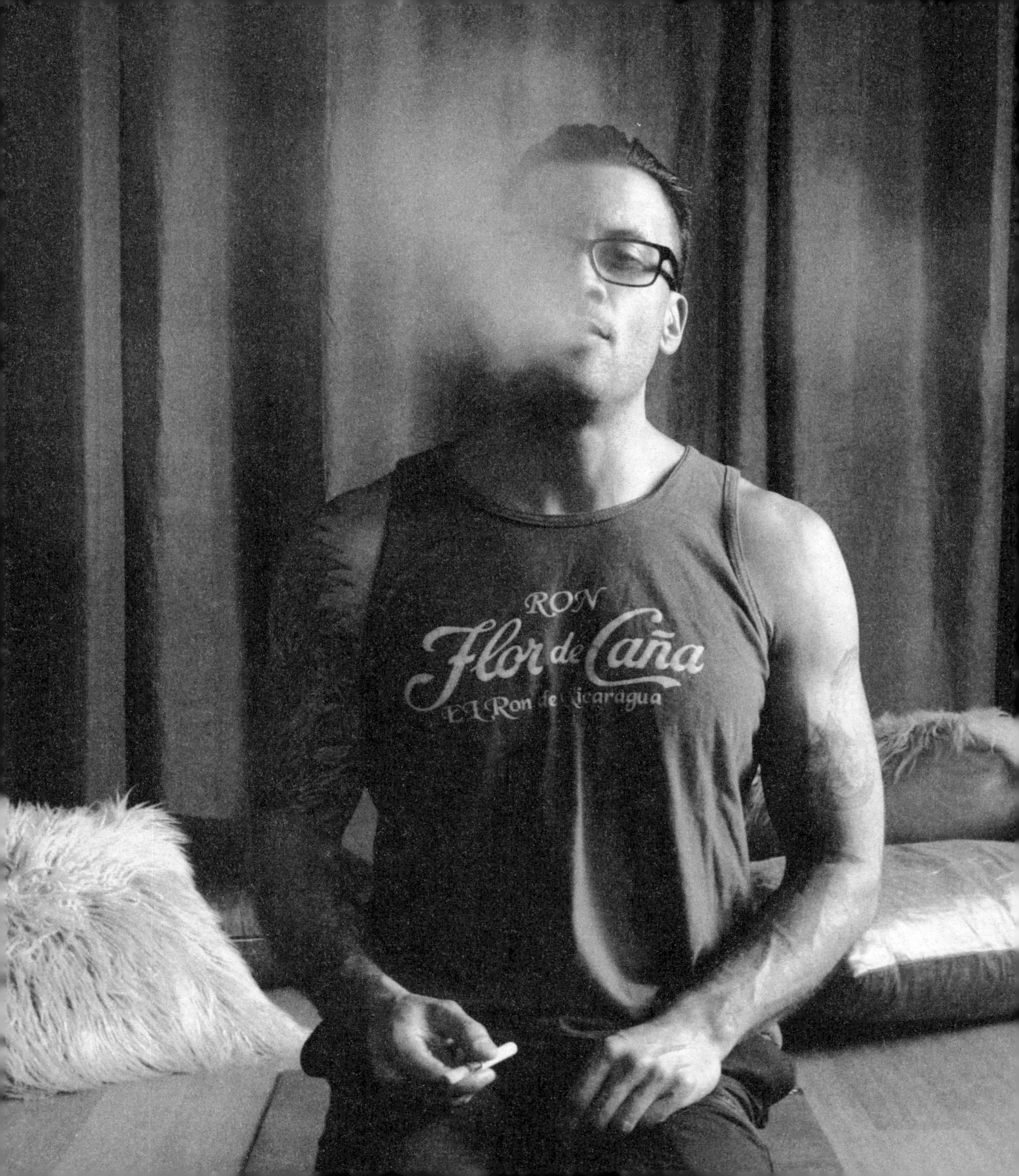

There is irrefutable evidence to suggest prehistoric use of cannabis by the ancient Sredni Stog (4500–3500 BCE) and Gonur (2000–1500 BCE) cultures of Ukraine and Turkmenistan. By the Iron Age, all of Europe was lit—evidence exists in Finland, Hungary, Denmark, the Czech Republic, and Germany.

Of all of antiquity's fellow travelers, though, the Pre-Colombian peoples of Central America deserve special mention for their whopping use of fifty-four species of hallucinogenic mushrooms. South American shamans from hunter-gatherer tribes that remained isolated into the twentieth century use roots, mushrooms, and vines for spiritual journeying; in recent years they've taken tens of thousands of Westerners on ayahuasca voyages in rituals that date back thousands of years.

The evidence is clear and unequivocal: human cultures across time and place have clearly used cannabis and other natural substances to expand consciousness. Some theorize that religion itself was born of the union between human neurons and psychotropic plants and animals.

But even if yogic history didn't lend enormous support for ganja-enhanced yoga, my direct experience is that the plant serves me. And that's all there is. On the first day of our yoga teacher training we were told that yoga is a personal science for the exploration and evolution of consciousness. Nothing that a teacher, guru, or sacred text tells you can mean more to you than your *direct experience*. With regard to your health, *you* need to be your own doctor; and spiritually, only *you* determine what feeds your soul.

In yoga, a guru is anything that dispels darkness and brings insight. It can be a situation, book, plant, or person.

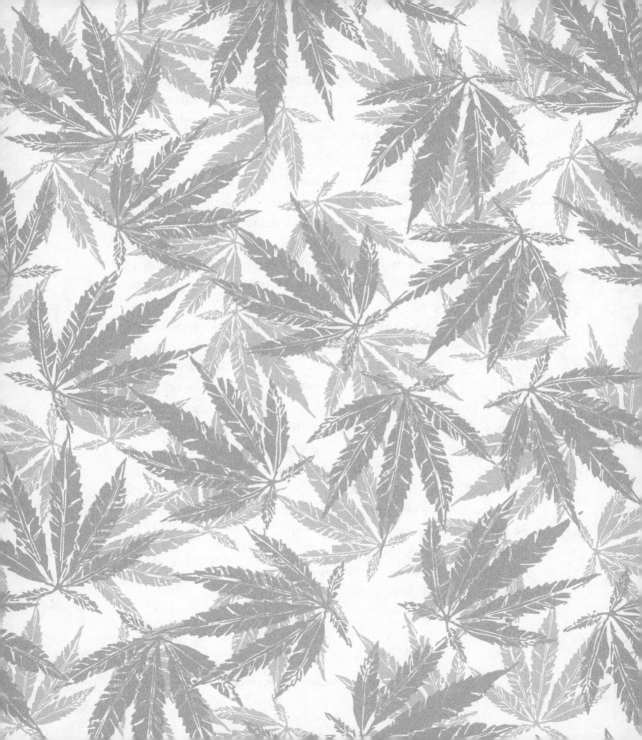

5

TANTRA YOGA IN AN (IMPOSSIBLE) NUTSHELL

NOW THAT YOU KNOW the history of stoney yoga, let's get into a little philosophy. There are two main branches of yoga: Tantra and Vedanta. As you'll see, Tantra is particularly suited to Ganja Yoga, so we'll be learning more about the theory behind it and the spiritual goals it aspires to.

Sacred Inclusivity

Tantra is about using our body, senses, sexuality, and feelings, our unique temperament and personality, and *all of our life experiences* to enhance our spiritual evolution. Tantra Yoga is designed to move us beyond disconnection, separation, and limitation.

There are many schools, philosophies, systems, and teachers of Tantra, but most would agree that Tantra does not support dualistic thinking; it does not view reality as composed of categories like pure and impure or even right and wrong (pretty much the opposite of what we're used to in the modern Western world). In Tantra, there is only what *is*. Acceptance and lack of dogma are foundational to this vastly misunderstood and deeply mysterious practice.

Vedanta, the other, newer branch of yoga, has a more dualistic view; it sees good and bad as moral absolutes. According to this form of yoga, the body and its sense delights and desires need to be actively transcended. According to the Vedantic approach, these "mundane" concerns distract us from what is real and really important, which is waking the spirit up and out of ego-identified consciousness. Although they share the same goal, the two forms of yoga take different approaches to get there.

Most popular yoga traditions based on Vedantic philosophy encourage extraordinarily rigorous physical and mental discipline. Two of the most popular Indian yoga teachers in the West, B. K. S. Iyengar (1918–2014) and K. Pattabhi Jois (1915–2009), are known for demanding abusive feats of purification from their students. According to the worldview of this form of yoga, cannabis use can only be a hindrance on the path.

> "According to Ayurveda, especially the tantric version, herbs are the embodiment of the living goddess. If applied properly, they release divine energies—to heal not only the physical aspect of our being, but the mental and spiritual aspects as well. . . . Herbs [also] play a significant role in the advanced practices of Tantra and kundalini yoga."
> —Pandit Rajmani Tigunait

Although Tantra agrees with the spiritual goal of awakening the consciousness out of lower, ego-centered ways of being into evolved, enlightened ones, it does not view the sensual side of our human experience as a distraction. It does not demand strict control. The philosophy of Tantra maintains that our human experiences, even though messy and ordinary, do not muddle our spiritual journey because *our human experiences are the spiritual journey.* Nice, right?

With this outlook, any moment—every experience, every craving, every emotion—can bring about liberation from limitation and ego, as long as we learn to be awake to life. Instead of avoiding what attracts us, we can choose to move into it with mindfulness and self-awareness and see if it leaves us feeling more spiritually connected.

Sex, Drugs, and Meditation

Some people think Tantra is all about sex, especially here in the United States, where the practice has been embraced by kinksters. This is because Tantra allows for and encourages us to use a vast array of tools in our daily human experience, *including sex.* But it is much more than that. Some forms of Tantra involve elaborate rituals; some see no purpose in ritual. Some tantrics use sexual energy; some are celibate. Although there are many different schools within Tantra, at its core it just wants us to wake up to the glorious awesomeness of life.

Seen through this lens, what we traditionally think of as vices may actually be sensory enhancers, catalysts for the tantric experience (when used mindfully). So in that vein, sex and drugs, if you don't mind my calling cannabis a drug for a moment, can be the fastest and most effective ways we humans have to wake up from the ego-driven, fear-based rat race of our day. According to Tantra, you should use them if you're called to and not use them if you aren't. In either case, be *intentional* and *self-aware*.

Sure, spending time in nature gets us there too. Yes, meditation works as well. But sex and cannabis are more immediate methods. In Tantra, you do not need to be anything other than what you are. If you do not have a secluded mountaintop ashram nearby to help you find your inner calm or get into an altered-state trance, no worries. You can instead intentionally use a natural, safe substance to quiet your racing mind or journey into your unconscious.

In the end, spirituality isn't about *what* we do, but *how* we do what we do. Whether we fast from food and pray for three days or roll a fatty before our yoga class, the quality of our spiritual experiences is determined by the consciousness we bring to our actions. If cannabis helps you to feel more connected to a loving higher purpose and takes you beyond limited ways of reacting to the world, then you are being served by your life choices, and you are practicing Tantra Yoga.

> How spiritual you are is more about your state of consciousness than the beliefs you hold.

You can still be a spiritual person, practice Tantra and other forms of yoga, and *not* consume cannabis, as I hope is clear. Many ways up the mountaintop! Each of us has our own spiritual path, and because it's so unique, we can never know where others are on their journey. The only thing we can fully grasp is our own path—what it looks like, how we feel, and what will get us where we want to be.

Of course, no matter the path to the mountaintop, certain practices ensure a smoother climb. The three most important things to remember for a successful Ganja Yoga experience are *mindfulness, safety,* and *intention.* Let's address them one by one, starting with mindfulness.

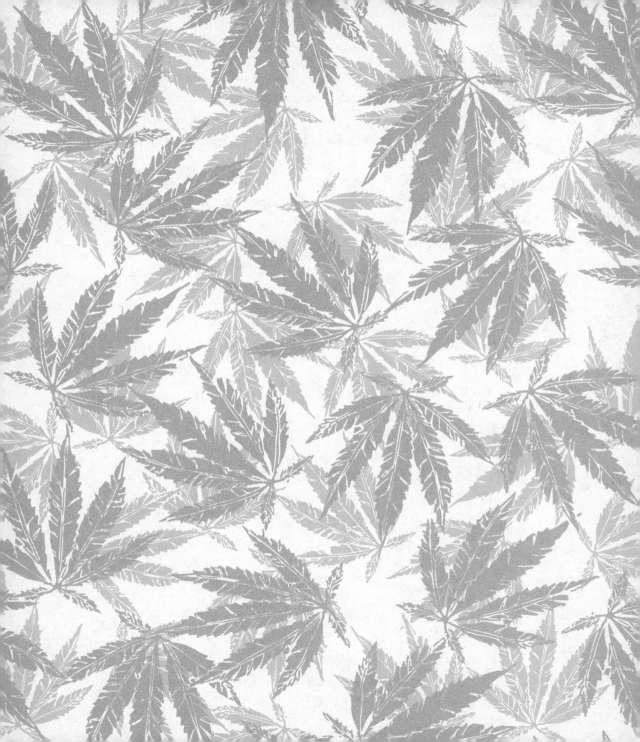

6

MEDICATED MINDFULNESS

PRESENCE AND *AWARENESS* are the words used to describe the yogic practice of cultivating the inner witness without judgment. In Buddhism, the word is *mindfulness*. Mindfulness is the practice of being fully in the present moment, fully awake and aware of it, instead of letting the mind wander to thoughts based on *what has happened* in the past or *what might happen* in the future.

Mindfulness is fairly popular right now, especially in the corporate world. From industry leaders like Google to back-end call centers, corporations are ensuring that their employees learn how to pay attention to the present moment, bringing less distraction and irritability and more well-being and harmony to the workday.

Instead of letting the mind flutter all over the place as it usually does, when we're mindful, we bring our attention to the present moment. Right as it is now. The whole of it or any part of it that we happen to notice. You can do it right now as you read. Just ask yourself, "What do I notice?"

Again and again, begin to notice sensation and impression, things inside, like thoughts and feelings, and things outside, like colors, sounds, and shapes. Notice what you like, what you don't like, and what you're neutral about. Notice your thinking about the noticing. Notice it all.

This practice brings greater metacognition, where you are increasingly aware of yourself as observer. "I am aware that I am angry" becomes the mindful moment, instead of simply, "I am angry," or worse, when you don't even know that you're angry and are expressing it in unhealthy ways.

So the first part of mindfulness is *choiceless awareness,* just letting your attention move like a butterfly from flower to flower in a relaxed way, not staying fixated on any one thing. One ten-second moment might look like: "I'm noticing my butt is getting numb," "I notice I want to end this conversation," "I notice those pretty shoes," and so on.

The second part of mindfulness is *acceptance.* Observations and impressions are simply noticed, then accepted without judgment or commentary. Sensations, people's words and behaviors, thoughts, even pain are part of this present moment. We bring a witnessing to it, and then we accept it and let it go, so we can be present to notice the next thing. Mindfulness is a practice that can be done anytime, and it will bring a peaceful calm to any situation.

Because mindfulness can be practiced in any and every moment of daily life, it has been called "meditation-in-motion." However, although mindfulness is a basic technique used in meditation, meditation practices themselves often go further. For example, in embodiment meditation you seek to become more in touch with body areas in order to relieve stress, and in concentration, or classic, meditation, you practice being single-pointed, focusing on an object like the breath, a mantra, a candle flame, or a series of instructions.

Mindfulness is awareness of the gestalt, having our attention on the whole of the experience without concentrating on one aspect. Though they have different goals and methodologies, mindfulness and meditation work cooperatively to strengthen one another. The more often we meditate, the more easily mindfulness arises. The more mindful we are, the deeper our meditations.

When people first start to shine the light of consciousness into their deep inner landscape many are surprised to see how much garbage exists in the mind. Luckily, in a very short period of time, the nonjudgmental self-awareness we develop from mindfulness makes us less emotionally reactive to our thoughts. Good thoughts, bad thoughts, amusing thoughts, horrible thoughts, creative thoughts, hateful thoughts—we see them all with less and less judgment, and we practice letting them come and go.

Over time, this practice helps us to be less reactive to others, able to see ourselves and other people with more patience and humor. We still feel the whole range of human emotions, but our emotions have less control over us. We're wiser, more aware of situations that upset, anger, and deplete us and, as a result, more able to address situations before they get out of hand.

Eventually, the practice of noticing and releasing the contents of your mind leads you to identify more with the awareness *behind* the thinking, not the thoughts or even the thinker. You begin to experience your body pains, personality preferences, thoughts, feelings, and opinions as transitory.

If your yoga goals are more about flexibility, relaxation, pain management, or a nice butt, Tantra Yoga says you are all good. I know that in our culture, not everyone is into the spiritual stuff. No matter what, mindful awareness is the foundation in yoga, the base for poses and breath practices.

While we do yoga poses, we practice holding a vivid awareness of the present moment as a gestalt, with a second layer of awareness on the sensations in the various body parts, chakras, or other subtle energy fields and the breath as it moves in the body. To do yoga poses or stretches without mindful attention is not yoga.

Mindfulness on and off the Mat

Mindfulness is not about clearing the mind. It's the attitude of having an open, accepting attitude toward whatever arises in your mind and the outside world. Cultivate it often. Notice all your reactions, desires, sensations, and thoughts. Notice the world around you, the colors, textures, sounds, and smells.

The more difficult you find it to stay present, the more mental tensions you probably have. It just means you haven't yet cultivated enough nervous system relaxation to soften the grip of an overwhelmed mind. Just keep practicing conscious relaxation and observation of the present moment, including your tensions, expectations, and assumptions. The relaxed alertness you patiently develop will slowly soften a constricted mind.

When one is truly aware of the present moment, there is a sense of clarity, lucidity, and ease. The more you notice in your life, the more richness you experience. The more you accept what you notice without judgment, the more ease and happiness you will feel. Mindfulness is something that each of us can experience at any time throughout the day, and once more, repetition of healthy habits allows us to create actual changes to our brain.

But let's not forget about the cannabis connection. The more mindfulness you practice, the more potent the effects of the cannabis. Energy flows where awareness goes. If you pay attention to the high, you'll amplify it, creating an even more open, expansive state of awareness. So stay present! Now, always, and especially as you toke.

And for those of you who are much more goal-oriented or coming to Ganja Yoga for practical reasons, I got you. Here are a few reasons, beyond the mystical, why mindfulness is beneficial.

Freedom from Stress

Like cannabis and yoga, mindfulness has both pragmatic and spiritual benefits. The main pragmatic benefit of mindfulness is that it brings freedom from the habit of responding to stress in ways that harm the body.

A stress reaction is a response to a mental or physical stressor that arouses the body's emergency resources. In modern life, our resources are continually tapped, leaving us suffering from irritability, anxiety, insomnia, depression, lowered immune response, fatigue, and high blood pressure.

The stressors we face are numerous. Fast-paced city life is stressful. We're constantly being sold to. We process more information in a day than most humans who ever existed received in a lifetime, and most of that information is negative news designed to draw outrage and clicks. These can be stressful to the body, even if we don't feel it consciously. Some other stressors that we barely register as such include constant social media notifications, feeling rushed, processed food, poor air quality, loud noises, artificial lighting, poor diet, overuse of stimulants or alcohol, too little movement, too little time outside, too little sleep, and far, far too much to do.

If this last paragraph makes you want to take a puff, I understand. *Go ahead; I'll wait.*

Although it can be stressful to think about all the toxic influences surrounding us, it's far more problematic to become accustomed to them, to accept them as the norm. By becoming invisible, they have even more power over us. But mindfulness makes us aware of these stressors. We become more sensitive to things that didn't even register on our observation radar before. Instead of suppressing the tension our imbalanced culture makes us feel, mindfulness helps us be aware of the unconscious stressors that move us from homeostasis, so we can take wise action. If possible, we leave the bar with a loud TV going, or take a much-needed nap, or practice yoga in a less busy studio so it's more relaxing.

Taking action to remove depleting environmental stressors is one way to reduce tension, but the more potent way is to become a master of your habitual stress reactions. When you habitually react to every stressor

THE RELAXATION RESPONSE

Cultivating the relaxation response allows you to improve your personal ability to encourage the brain to release chemicals that relax the muscles, increase blood flow to the organs, and slow a busy mind. There are many methods in the yoga tradition and beyond. Regular engagement of the relaxation response results in less stress and more well-being. Learning how to elicit relaxation at will is one of the most valuable things we can do in life.

Spend some quiet time every day tapping inward to connect to yourself. Be aware of yourself relaxing. Even a few minutes will bring immense results!

as though it's an emergency (as most of us do at the physical and biochemical level), you tax the adrenal glands, and they become hyperactive and less functional, squirting cortisol with little provocation and getting you into a cycle of more easily triggered stress responses.

Constant stress decreases the power of your immune system. It makes it hard to sleep. It makes it hard to make rational choices. New research in the United Kingdom draws a strong linear correlation between psychological distress and premature killers like cancer, heart disease, and even car accidents. Mindfulness changes your response to stress, so stressors don't harm your health.

When you practice keeping the mind in the present moment and when you use cannabis to heighten this self-awareness, you're less easily conditioned to act as you did in the past. You have more clarity, objectivity, and wisdom instead of being animated by your every desire and fear like a puppet or inflating each conflict or irritation into an emergency. Awareness allows you to go through life with authentic responses instead of habitual reactions. You're able to respond to each new difficult situation, which may indeed be stressful, from your center. If the goal of yoga is spiritual liberation, the freedom from stress that mindfulness brings is a taste of that, available to everyone at any time.

Freedom from Pain

The simplest form of learning occurs through constant repetition. When the same bodily actions are done over and over again—if we repeatedly stand, sit, walk, drive, or even practice yoga in a certain way—the body becomes accustomed to the repeated behavior and the tissues are gradually changed to make it easier to do.

Your body will unconsciously adapt to any posture or movement you use regularly, whether it is a helpful adaptation or not. If you sit a lot, your calves and hamstring muscle fibers will *physically shorten* to help you sit more. If you spend a lot of time in front of a screen, head forward, lower back rounding, shoulders slumped, your body gets used to that position because it's what it thinks you want. Although this adaptation may make sitting and texting easy, when it's time to walk or do anything else, your short, tight muscles will cause pressure on the joints, leading to inflammation and pain.

PAIN ISN'T WHAT YOU THINK

Science is teaching us a new understanding of pain. Fascinating new studies have shown that cues sent from an injury site are not "pain," as we'd previously thought, but rather a simple message to indicate to the brain that something might be wrong. In a split second, the brain takes this message, say, that you stubbed your toe, along with all the other incoming messages it is receiving about the environment, to decide if the tissue damage will be felt as pain.

The associations your brain makes about the injury and your emotional state when your brain gets the warning both impact whether the brain perceives pain. Pain is not an input to the brain from the injury site; it is a response from the brain that the injury needs to be attended to. In moments of running for our lives or moving to save the lives of others, the brain decides that even severe tissue damage does not need to be prioritized, and we don't feel pain until later, when we're safely at rest. Likewise, when athletes are extremely committed to the sport they're playing, injuries are usually felt only after the game is over.

The link between tissue damage and pain is actually weak. Many people have pain from body parts they no longer even have, and many others experience no pain from injuries that can be seen medically. Stress, anxiety, and depression all impact the brain's creation of pain.

Whether you've been diagnosed with tissue damage or not, if you are experiencing pain, the best way to handle it is to manage your stress, anxiety, and depression. Don't let your pain make you worry about pain, because that causes more pain. Just be with pain, mindfully accepting it, even if it hurts.

Be compassionate with yourself, find pleasure in your body where you can, and hang in there.

Think of how your body responds every time your phone beeps. What shape does it take? What shape does it take as you rush to cross the street on time? What's your posture when a deadline looms? The "stressors" are normal experiences in our ordinary world, but if they happen often enough, your body prepares for the constant triggering and remains contracted, ready for action. Then the state of habitual contraction becomes "normal," and we're left with short muscles, tightness, tension, pain, and a reduced ability to breathe deeply or cycle nutrition and lymph. This is why many of us have pain or are unable to relax our tight, stiff body.

No more. Mindfulness helps us to become aware of the habitually contracted spots we have in the body, so we can bring more, different, or less movement to them. Maybe we decide all texting will be done standing up, to lengthen the leg muscles. Maybe we start to realize we always sit in the same posture when watching TV and change it up. Maybe we add dancing to our jogging routine. Maybe we do work calls while walking, instead of in front of a screen. The ways we can de-stress the body are endless and worth pursuing, no matter your age or mobility level.

The practice of mindfulness isn't just naked awareness, but noticing the things that make us feel better or worse. As we observe and accept what is, we can then choose the things that are more beneficial.

Mindfulness Practice

It bears repeating: mindfulness can be practiced anytime. It is really just a matter of asking, "What do I notice, inside and outside?" and then "being with" (accepting) whatever it is that you notice.

Ask the question again and again. "I'm noticing that the last few minutes I've been really distracted from work because I'm thinking about dinner." "I observe that my spine is rounded as I type." "I am aware of myself judging the person on the next mat over because she is breathing really loudly." And so on. We don't get emotionally reactive about what we notice, but if it isn't serving us and we are able to, we change it.

Just as mindfulness helps us release habitual patterns of muscular contraction and emotional reactivity, it also brings more appreciation of the present moment. "I am aware of the pretty color of paint in this room." "I'm noticing my wife's soft hand in mine." Giving our full attention to someone is one of the best gifts we can give. And honoring life, showing up for our own life, is one of the best gifts we can give to ourselves. Of course, if the present moment is delicious, as it often is during yoga, sex, and time in nature, then it's even easier to stay present. After some time, staying present occurs more and more often, so that you're able to be mindful of and even appreciate life's more mundane moments.

Every time we bring awareness to the way we move, think, and act, we set a more solid foundation for a healthier life. Mindfulness is not an effort to suppress the inner restlessness of the mind, but a nonjudgmental curiosity about it, a willingness to observe it as it happens. There's good reason why mindfulness is so huge right now. It's powerful. I have found that my own life has undergone a radical transformation as a result of mindfulness practice. Take a moment to look up from the page right now and notice five things around you and five things within you.

Now, want to make mindfulness even more captivating? *Just add weed.*

GET HIGH THE MINDFUL WAY

For this mindful toking practice, have everything you need handy for a good high. I recommend vaping (inhaling vaporized cannabis), so you can really savor the flavor and aroma. If possible, have more than one strain available to vape, so you can bring more sensitivity to the differences in taste between strains. Newbies: If you have never heard of vaping before and are scratching your head about strains, we'll break it down in Chapters 9 and 10.

All right. Ready?

Sustain an alert, flexible, and focused attention when practicing mindfulness. You are *alert* and awake, but at the same time you are as relaxed as you can be. You are *flexible,* taking from the variety of sensory experiences and impressions that occur all the time. Sometimes you'll notice the taste of the vape or the feeling of your breath; sometimes it will be the music, or a car going by. Your attention is *focused* on the present moment, returning to any aspect of it whenever you find your mind wandering off to thoughts.

Relaxation is not the goal, but an eventual outcome of mindfulness. If there's pain or tension, be with it. Sometimes noticing is simply a matter of "I am aware that I'm feeling really grumpy and not in the mood for this right now." The only goal of mindfulness is to expand the awareness.

1. With all this in mind, begin to get high without doing anything else at the same time. Put down your phone. As you begin to ingest the cannabis, notice whatever you notice, without judgment or expectation. Keep doing that, greeting each sensation and impression with awareness and curiosity. Pay particular attention to the taste of each strain.

2. Take a moment to notice the following things: a sound, a feeling in the body, the breath. Repeat. Usually mindfulness is "choiceless" awareness, letting whatever you notice be what you notice, but for beginners it's good to explore the different categories of things there are to notice. Do two or three rounds of this and then let the awareness of the present moment be free so it can take in the whole or other finer details.

3. Enjoy it! Bringing awareness to the present moment deepens the richness of it. Time moves more slowly; you get to savor. However, as you notice things in the moment, you may also begin to notice things inside your head that you don't necessarily like. Be a silent witness to the thoughts you observe. Instead of beating yourself up for what you find when you shine the light of awareness inside your mind, learn to accept your dark thoughts and shadow aspects. Allow them to integrate them as a part of you—a part of being human—and they'll eventually transform.

4. Continue to practice mindfulness after the consumption experience is over. Be mindful of being high. And whenever you can throughout your day, consciously relax your body and check in with yourself, noticing your thoughts, your mood, your judgments, your reactions, and all your impressions, with acceptance.

Bring this mindfulness into your daily life, for it is an "anytime, all the time" practice.

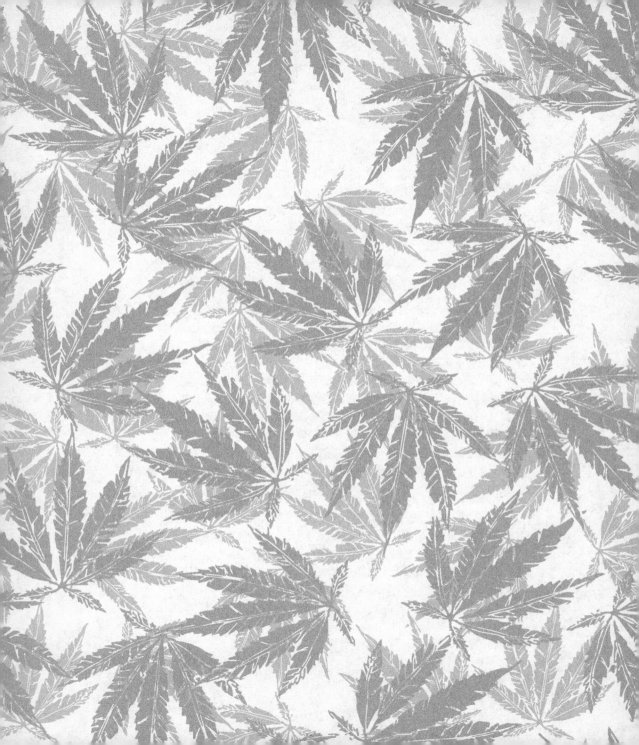

7

SAFE STONERS

WHEN I TELL PEOPLE THAT I teach cannabis-enhanced yoga, I usually get a positive response, something like, "Far out, man. I get high before class all the time!" or "Neat. What strains are best?"

The rare time a concern does get raised, it's always about safety. The concerned person is probably projecting an internalized stereotypical stoner image onto me and my students: bleary, red, half-closed eyes; slow response time; clumsy; somewhat stupid. But this is not at all what I see when I look around my classroom on Wednesday and

Thursday nights in San Francisco. Sure, there are a few hippie types, but there are just as many smart techies, health-minded folks, and CEOs. There are moms, retirees, and loving couples (even people on awesome first dates!).

The thing is, as a culture, we don't yet have a nuanced picture of cannabis because of a century of misinformation and propaganda. More and more people are coming out of the closet to show that we can be intelligent, successful stoners, but public perception will take a long time to change. I'm okay with that, glad to be a part of the cultural redefinition!

However, when it comes to safety, I actually do have a bone to pick. Ironically, however, it's not with the ganja part of the practice.

A number of reports from the last five to ten years are beginning to show soft-tissue and joint injuries that *came from practicing yoga*. Yep, you read right. More and more well-respected teachers, like Diane Bruni from Toronto, have come forth to share how they suffered injuries as a result of their (sober) yoga practice. These revelations of course shocked the yoga community. After all, we've been prescribing yoga practices to bring *relief* from nearly every type of health ailment a person could have, and to now find that it can sometimes be the *cause* of our pain . . .

Safety Issues

Thankfully, many of the safety issues related to yoga can be eliminated with information and self-awareness. Whether you're practicing sober or enhancing with cannabis, it is your job, and your job only, to ensure you're treating your body right while doing yoga. Here are some of the things you may be doing wrong—and easy fixes for each problem.

OVERSTRETCHING

Many people, yoga teachers included, do not realize that tightness, or lack of range of motion, in a joint is usually *not related to muscle length*. When we can't stretch farther in a pose, oftentimes it isn't our short muscles limiting the range, but rather our *nervous system putting the kibosh on movements that take the joints into positions we don't put them in regularly*. This is called the *stretch reflex*.

When people are given anesthesia, they are able to perform stretches they were unable to do before. This means it isn't hamstring shortness preventing you from moving the tailbone higher in Downward Dog, but your nervous system resisting a new (read: scary) movement that could cause injury. Because of our limited daily movement habits, that stretch feels outside our movement range. (Thanks for lookin' out, nervous system!)

The problem is that we, as a highly sedentary culture, don't put our bodies into very many different shapes, so that our wise nervous system develops increased intolerance for new movements. *The less we move, the less we can move*. Read that sentence again and then take a ten-second stretch break . . .

Hi, welcome back.

Now get this. When we ignore our nervous system and overstretch in yoga, the muscles we're trying to lengthen, like the hamstrings in Downward Dog, actually respond to the nervous system intolerance by contracting *against* the stretch. That means when we push ourselves in yoga, our muscles end up *more* contracted than before the practice. Ouch.

> Your body is the temple for your soul. Keep it in good condition.

Our culture doesn't like to hear this, but "more" is not always better. "More" means we end up shorter and tighter, not longer and freer. Keep this in mind the next time you feel the sensation of tightness as you practice. Instead of pushing the tissues to where you think they should be, *gently* coax yourself, *over a span of time*, into greater ranges of motion in the places you feel limited, stiff, tight, and sore. This respects your body's hardware (the tissues) and the software (the nervous system). Once more, the mantra is, "Don't overstretch!"

NOT KNOWING THE DIFFERENCE BETWEEN PAIN AND SENSATION

Another way we might hurt ourselves in yoga, whether sober or enhanced with cannabis, is ignoring our pain cues. Sensation is a part of being embodied and mindful. It's a part of being human. Sensation can become strong when we move the body into shapes it doesn't usually take. Stretching can feel good, weird, even slightly intense, but there should never, ever, be anything even close to pain.

Notice if you are becoming tense in your body or mind as a result of the poses. Observe if you're clenching or wincing or if your breathing is compromised. These are markers that you might be ignoring pain signals. Be sure to breathe deeply through the nose in each pose. If you can't, back off the stretch. And at any time in your practice, feel free to back off from the instruction and rest, even when in a conventional yoga studio class where everyone else is working hard. Respect your body and over time you'll develop open communication

> Yoga is not about flexibility, stretching, or moving deeper into a posture.
>
> Yoga is a way of living that encourages mindful moving, breathing, thinking, and being.

with it, so you will immediately know if you would be better served by doing something else.

NOT REALIZING WHAT WE CAN AND CANNOT DO

Our sedentary, stressful lifestyle can make us susceptible to yoga injuries. Many of us sit in the same general posture throughout the day: driving, eating, working at the computer, playing on our phones, watching TV. As a result, we carry a tremendous amount of tension through the neck and shoulders. As *Yoga Journal* suggests, if we then go to a yoga class with lots of repetitions of Chaturanga Dandasana, where we move from a push-up straight down to the floor several times, this can place even more stress on the vulnerable joints and cause injury, even if our alignment is perfect (which, let's face it, is often not the case).

Think about the movements you do a lot already in day-to-day life and find a restorative yoga practice that *balances* your lifestyle. Make a point to move your body in new positions as often as you can throughout the day and mix up your yoga routine to get as many joint positions as possible. Also, avoid doing the same yoga sequence over and over again, which can wreak havoc on vulnerable joints.

Most important, instead of trusting that all poses are for all people and all poses should be done however many times the teacher says or for however long she says, consider your unique body's imbalances. There are countless modifications and variations if the traditional postures are not working for you. Don't be too cool to use a yoga block or strap to maintain good

> Remember, your yoga practice is "you time," where you can let go of wondering what the teacher or the rest of the class thinks.

alignment, and if you're not sure how, do some research or consult a private teacher.

Knowing what we can and cannot do brings a sense of acceptance and humbleness. It's great for the soul.

ZONING OUT

This cautionary note encapsulates the first three. If you don't zone out, if you are practicing the art of mindfulness, you won't overstretch, ignore pain cues, or blindly follow your yoga teacher. Remember, yoga is *mental* as much as it is physical.

And finally . . .

The Ego: The Number-One Cause of Yoga Injury

Yang is a Chinese word that describes the exterior, directed, and forceful aspects of reality. The internal, non-goal-oriented, and receptive aspects of life are called *yin*.

Most people's yoga practice, and in fact our entire Western culture, is heavily *yang*. We think of yoga as something to be *performed,* not something you can *feel.* We are a visual culture, an accomplishment-based culture. Instagram and social-media celebrities thrill us with athletic, impossible-seeming poses, reinforcing our in-class fixation on how we *look*. As such, the practice has become extraordinarily body-oriented in the past thirty years, with a focus not only on posturing (as opposed to meditation and breathing), but also on the attainment of challenging and visually interesting postures.

Caring for the body as a sacred vessel is the first principle of yoga. *Expanding consciousness to awaken to our fullest potential* is the second.

Practice the art of focusing inward, slowing down, and staying present. If you're able to practice these, even a little bit, then you can do yoga, and if you're able to practice these while high on cannabis, then you can do Ganja Yoga. The specific postures, which were originally designed to allow us to sit in meditation for longer periods, are icing on the cake. Something to remember in our visual, competitive culture.

I get it, these poses look cooler on social media. But when we bring our Western acquisitiveness to yoga, we usually end up overdoing it.

By definition, yoga is about the spiritual and psychological rewards of patience, which takes a lifetime of practice. Regardless of one's beliefs or goals, Ganja Yoga is about cultivating balance and harmony, not perfecting an arm balance or going farther into a pose than the person on the next mat.

If your ego wants to compete against other students, or against what you were able to do last week, or against what you think you *should* be able to do, bring in the element of mindfulness. Make that the most important part of your practice. Notice, with compassion, your urge to extend beyond your threshold. Be with it. *Breathe into it.* Practice seeing the desire to push yourself beyond your edge as it arises, without giving in to it. Notice frustrations and self-judgments that come up, cultural conditioning you may have absorbed that causes you to focus on poses that look cool.

If the result feels like a more "boring" yoga practice, be with that, especially if you have many years of yoga practice under your belt. Development in yoga consists of deepening your somatic awareness and self-acceptance, not attaining shapes.

Cultivating Beginner's Mind

How do simple poses like the Table Pose or the Child Pose feel when your consciousness is present the entire time? How does a basic pose change when your movements are enhanced by plant medicine? How is your practice altered when you're in a more sensitive, suggestible state? What happens when you slow down? When you do less?

When students request more intermediate poses, I ask them whether they've managed to keep their minds steady and calm through the basic postures, and if not, there's no need to graduate to harder-looking stuff. Sure, I sometimes throw in a challenging pose; it's fun, and you get a sense of accomplishment from mastering something you weren't able to do before. But the real accomplishment of yoga, and one that is truly safe, is the psychological and spiritual development you do *inside,* where no one can see it.

If you love your yoga physically challenging, you're able to ensure good alignment, and you can practice with restraint and gentleness, more power to you for either sober or enhanced practice! Never forget, though, how completely necessary relaxation is for health and longevity in this frantic time. Relaxation is a basic human need, not a luxury. Be sure to balance your energizing, powerful yoga practice with lots of relaxing *yin* experiences to ensure you attain the most benefit.

Although it's just not humanly possible to prevent all injuries, keeping these points in mind will go a long way to ensuring a safe yoga practice, whether sober or enhanced with ganja. It all goes back to mindfulness and self-kindness. In the chapter on postures, we'll go into actual alignment points specific to each pose. It is my life's work to ensure physical safety when my students are in altered states, and my detailed instructions have their foundation in biomechanics and injury prevention.

If you are still wondering about safety as it relates to cannabis, don't worry. I'll walk you through the best ways to consume in Chapter 9. In the meantime, remember that the most important safety precaution in Ganja Yoga is body awareness.

KEEP IT SAFE

1. To let the nervous system *allow* the muscles to lengthen, it's important to go slow in yoga, building toward a deeper stretch within the pose itself. For example, as you take your first Downward Dog, move around in it, get used to it, come out of it and then go back into it, warming up the body and playing around before eventually finding the "full expression" of the pose.

2. Do more intense stretches toward the end of the yoga session, when the nervous system has been convinced it is okay to move beyond the joint ranges you go into in your day-to-day.

3. Move frequently to change up habitual positions, and drink a lot of fluids so your connective tissues don't "freeze up" as much. Give yourself permission to take plenty of movement and stretching breaks throughout the day.

4. While practicing Ganja Yoga, do stretches and poses that put your body into shapes that are different from those of your daily routine. Often have your neck forward to look at your phone? Try poses where you pull your ears so they're more over the shoulders to give the neck a break. Often sitting with the knees bent? Give the calves a chance to lengthen with a Downward Dog or calf stretch.

5. Cultivate patience. Graduate to harder poses over the course of many weeks, months, and years. There is no destination or final pose to accomplish, only the journey of slowly opening and feeling your body.

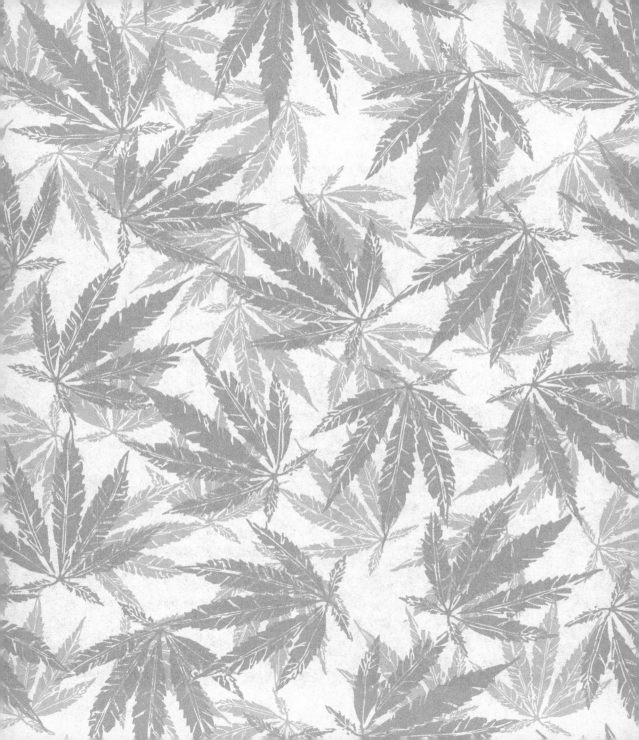

8

INTENTION SETTING

YOGA AND CANNABIS produce altered states of consciousness on their own, and as you know they work even more powerfully when combined. Both tools quiet the mind-set fashioned from the linear, goal-oriented, socially conditioned experiences of daily life, the stuff of muggles, production and consumption, which so often leaves us feeling as though we are the ones being consumed. With yoga and cannabis, the subtle yet remarkable experiences of fully occupying a body and engaging a relaxed mind become more apparent. We feel *creative, magical, inspired, turned-on, present, satisfied.*

When cannabis and yoga are used in an *intentional* way, the expanded mental, emotional, psychological, and spiritual states are even more pronounced. To be intentional means to have a desire—a want, need, or wish—and to invite the experience at hand to fulfill this intention. When we're intentional with our cannabis consumption, we ask, "Why am I consuming this?" or "What would I like from this?" Knowing where we are and where we would like to be brings more mindfulness, reverence, and even a sense of magic to the stoned experience.

Sometimes I want to focus extra attention on being easy on myself, so I bring the intention of gentleness to that yoga practice. At other times, when I have more energy and less need for nurturing, my intention is to do a few more strength-based poses than my lazy ass would like. Sometimes I wish for clarity about a situation and intentionally choose a focusing meditation and a strain of cannabis that provides a cerebral, mood-elevating high, matching my tools to my intentions.

As you check in with what you intend for the session, also check with yourself to make sure you have no other responsibilities you're neglecting that could interfere with your high. Especially if you're new to cannabis, try trippin' only on nights when you don't have a big meeting with the boss the next morning.

To help yourself make your intention a reality, turn your ringer off and in fact put your phone far, far away. What else do you need? A candle? Soft music? You could even prepare a snack for later, since preventative self-care is the best medicine.

Although the endocannabinoid system works on a biological level regardless of our intention, we can enhance the physiological benefits with the power of our intention.

UTILIZE THE HIGH!

Set your intention by asking yourself:

1. "Where am I at right now?" (Am I tired? In pain? Or feeling chill and easygoing?)

2. "What do I want from this experience?" (Do you want to feel energized? Connected? Free of pain?)

3. "Is now a good time to get high?" (Do I have any responsibilities I need to take care of? How long can I be altered for?)

4. "How can I utilize the cannabis to get that need met?" (Which method shall I use? How can I set the space? What kind of props/toys, music, and lighting would enhance the experience?)

5. "What kind of ritual can I create for additional potency?"

The Lost Art of Ritual

The use of ceremony has been lost in most of the modern world, even in most yoga studio environments. For those of us who were forced to perform empty rituals as part of our religious upbringing, we can rightly be suspicious of the word.

However, when creating the intention for a spiritual cannabis experience or an altered state of consciousness, understand that "sacredness" is whatever *you* make meaningful or important. "Ritual" is whatever you want it to be. As long as your mind is present and the intention is there to create nonordinary, spiritual space, that is all that needs to be done.

MAKING OBJECTS SACRED

Whenever you ascribe spiritual meaning to something, it becomes a sacred thing. At the top of your mat, place crystals and gemstones, if they speak to you, or any object that evokes a positive feeling, like a photograph or pretty leaf. To imbue it with sacred feeling, hold it in your hand for a moment as you set your intention for the high or the yoga practice. Using a sentence, phrase, or word, speak your intention aloud or simply think it. By placing the object at the top of your yoga mat, you'll remind yourself of your intention and be more likely to have the experience you desire.

Sometimes it's just a matter of clearing off the coffee table and lighting some incense before blazing, setting a sacred object at the top of your mat, or doing a closed-eye visualization of a symbol or something from nature before starting your poses.

The Ganja Yoga ritual can be anything you want, or nothing at all. If you're called to use cannabis, invite a sense of reverence for it before smoking. Light candles to create a sacred space (space different from your usual hangout space), burn some incense, or even repeat a Sanskrit incantation. You can use *Bhava na sana hridayam* (bah-vah nah sah-nah hree-dye-yahm), which means, "May this cannabis be a blessing to my heart," or evoke Shiva, the Lord of Ganja, with *Om namah Shivaya* (ohm nah-mah shee-vye-yah).

As you make up your own ritual, know that for thousands of years, many gurus and babas have been ritualistically using cannabis for yoga practice, as you are here. You might evoke them, call in their wisdom and energy, or send a mental prayer of gratitude for them and for the plant.

Perhaps you send a blessing of thanks to the farmers. If it feels more right to connect to the feminine energy of the plant, you might incorporate it into a form of Goddess worship.

Your ritual might be an affirmation that speaks to your intention; phrase it as though it's already true in the present tense. A good one for Ganja Yoga is, "My body is strong, balanced, and relaxed." Your ritual might be very basic, just a few deep breaths before inviting the sacred medicine into your body. Whatever you do, when it's time to consume, treat the cannabis sacredly, ingesting it with conscious awareness. As you move into practice, keep this intention and sacred attitude.

Only the female cannabis plants are used (males are bred out). That is our cue to use cannabis to intentionally blend our unique spiritual path with feminism and respect for women and mothers everywhere, a modern form of Goddess worship.

Even if your yoga goals are more mundane than transformation, it's important to believe that any spiritual, psychological, or physical goal you have for yourself is possible. After all, the first requirement to meet any goal is a belief that the goal is possible to attain. Don't worry if you want to touch your toes or have a better bum. Some of us come to yoga for the Zen of it and others don't. The Ganja Yoga guru (Shiva) says, "Judge not your fellow yogis" and then passes the blunt your way.

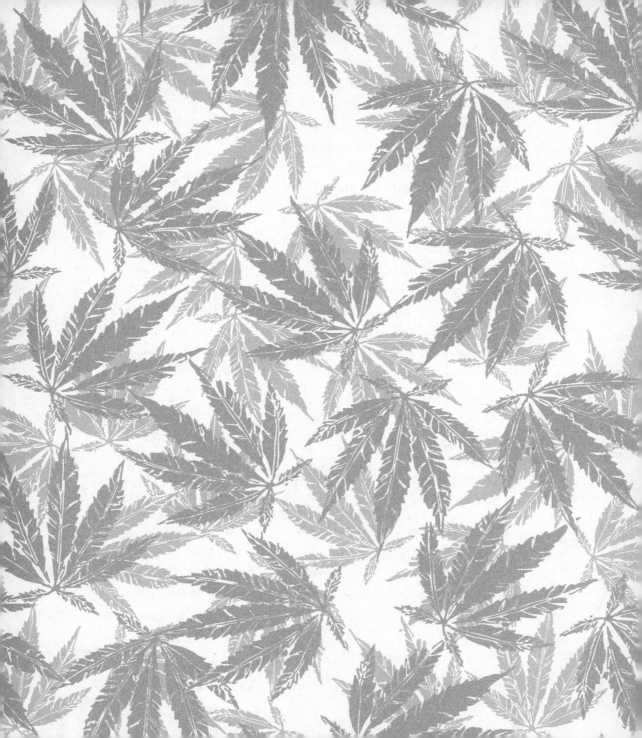

9

HOW TO ENHANCE:
Methods of Consumption

THERE ARE MANY WAYS we can use cannabis, and each provides a unique experience. It can be intimidating to learn new methods, but with such a rich world out there, it is worth digging in.

Different strains of cannabis have different ratios of THC and CBD along with various amounts of up to eighty-three other cannabinoids; each strain therefore has its own cannabinoid profile. But this isn't the only consideration that a ganja yogi has to make when choosing a strain. Before we consider the methods, we need to take an unexpected journey into the delicious world of terpenes.

89

Terpenes: The Flavor Factor

Ever notice how some weed smells like citrus, berries, musky cheese, diesel gasoline, or a pine forest? *Terpenes* are the aromatic essential oils that give each cannabis strain its distinctive fragrance and flavor. A variety of other plants, herbs, fruits, vegetables, and trees also contain terpenes.

Terpenes are thought to protect plants by deterring herbivores or to help in procreation by drawing pollinators and herbivores that spread pollen and seeds.

A certain strain of cannabis can express many terpenes at once, creating a complex and unique terpene profile. When various terpene profiles are combined with the many different cannabinoid profiles, thousands of unique cannabis strains can be created. As we'll see, it's this variety of terpenes—many of which have an active impact on the brain chemistry—that makes "cannabis" not one monolithic drug, but instead a whole class of substances that have different physiological and psychotropic effects.

Over one hundred different terpenes have been identified in the cannabis plant. Along with providing the sensual element of

In recent years, as terpenes have come to be recognized as important parts of the taste and medicinal effect of cannabis, many suppliers began adding terpenes from other plants to vape cartridges to enhance the effect. But a recent study in Brazil may herald a change back to strain-specific profiles, finding that the addition of a noncannabis-derived terpene did more harm than good. Definitely something to be aware of as you select your terpene-tasty vape pens.

sniffing some good bud before you blaze and savoring the lingering taste on the palette as you exhale, terps offer an array of proven health benefits. Some terpenes can boost serotonin and GABA to create feelings of happiness and relaxation, while others boost dopamine and norepinephrine. Some terpenes and terpene combinations have been shown to be especially good for relieving stress, while others help with sleep or bring mental clarity. Some liken the range and variation in terpenes to those of wine: connoisseurs explore the nose and palette of different varietals and learn the art of pairing for maximum pleasure.

Medical research on cannabis has been so focused on cannabinoids (not to mention, so late to the game!), we don't yet know much about terps, but we do know that they modulate our body's interaction with cannabinoids by also binding to endocannabinoid receptor sites and affecting the chemical output. Terpenes enhance the therapeutic and psychoactive effect of cannabinoids.

Again, it's the whole-plant entourage effect that comes into play, giving us various strains of this holistic medicine, each with a specific aroma and effect.

Common Terpenes

Here are some of the most common terpenes found in cannabis. As you sample them, see if you can begin to taste and smell the unique flavors and feel any specific healing effects.

PINENE

One of the most common terpenes is pinene, which is also found in conifer trees, rosemary, and orange peels. This pine-smelling compound has been shown to be a bronchodilator, helping people with breathing conditions. Ever been invigorated by the fresh air in a mountain pine forest? Pinene was there to open up your lungs. It has also been shown to be an anti-inflammatory, antibacterial, analgesic (painkiller), antioxidant, and antibiotic as well as a memory aid and antidepressant. Sour Diesel and Blue Dream are strains that have a lot of pinene.

MYRCENE

A musky-smelling terp, myrcene is present in hops and numerous cannabis varietals, especially strong indicas. It provides a sedative effect and has been shown to be a muscle relaxant, analgesic (painkiller), and anti-inflammatory, giving a deep "couchlock" experience. Try Purple Kush or Super Silver Haze for myrcene.

LINALOOL

Also found in lavender, linalool has anesthetic, analgesic, anticonvulsant, and anxiolytic (anti-anxiety) properties. One study found that linalool reduces carcinogenic lung inflammation caused by tobacco smoke, suggesting that it likely does the same for cannabis smoke. Get some ganja with the word "purple" in the title for a high chance at scoring some linalool.

LIMONENE

An essential oil also found in lemons, limonene has been shown to improve mood, offering anti-anxiety and antidepressant qualities. It can lower cholesterol and relieve heartburn and acid reflux. Limonene also has some extremely intriguing anticancer properties. Strains that smell like citrus include Lemon Haze and OG Kush.

Puff like a Pro

THE BEST WAYS TO ENSURE A ROBUST ENDOCANNABINOID SYSTEM INCLUDE:

- Smoking
- Vaping
- Edibles
- Tinctures
- Topicals
- Concentrates

The six main methods of consumption are below, with tips and techniques for getting the best cannabinoid and terpene experience. If you're a beginner, have a read, notice which methods appeal to you, and start with those.

SMOKING

People have been burning dried plant matter and inhaling the smoke for thousands of years, usually in connection with religious or social rituals. Whether you prefer a joint or pipe, this is very different from the modern habit of blindly going through a pack of cigarettes a day.

There is no link between cannabis and lung cancer, even for heavy smokers.

PROS	CONS
Smoking has a nice fast onset for those ready to get to business. It's easy and intuitive.	Smoking anything, even something noncarcinogenic like cannabis, can have potential negative health consequences, because the combustion of any plant matter produces harmful compounds.
It's clear how high you are, so you can titrate (dose) more accurately than with other methods.	
It is an ancient and highly sensory experience that connects us to the element of fire.	Burning your cannabis destroys many of the flavorful and healing terpenes, which are needed for the full entourage effect.
It feels more social and badass sexy to pass a joint than a vape.	

Tips

- To reduce exposure to smoke, don't hold the toke in! Draw one or two puffs deep into your lungs (do not rest the smoke in the throat), and then take an optional sip of fresh air as well to cool the smoke. Exhale immediately.

- Smoke higher-potency products, so you'll inhale fewer combustible irritants.

- When you directly apply a flame to the cannabis, more toxic compounds are produced and more cannabinoids and terpenes are lost. Make a point to "cherry" your joint or pipe instead of repeatedly lighting it.

- A hemp wick is a long string of hemp dipped in beeswax and often wrapped around a lighter. You light the hemp and use that flame to light your pipe or doobie; it provides cooler combustion than a lighter, with not even a trace amount of noxious lighter fluid! It you prefer a lighter, flick it on first and then apply it to your doobie or bowl, so you aren't slurping up butane as well, and use as little flame as you can.

- Use thin, natural, bleach-free papers for your joints, ideally ones made of hemp.

- Learn to roll your own joints, since prerolls are often made from lesser-quality "shake" (cannabis trimmings that contain less potent flowers and some leaves). Make a filter from a small roll of cardboard.

- Use only glass pipes, and clean them often by soaking them in a mix of rubbing alcohol, salt, and dish soap; use an opened paper clip to pull gunk out of the mouthpiece as needed. If you use rubbing alcohol to clean your paraphernalia, be sure to rinse any residue, and make sure your pipe is completely dry before toking.

- What little research there is on methods of cannabis ingestion indicates that water will filter some of the healing cannabinoids, leaving an even greater ratio of tar and particulate matter to cannabinoids, requiring you to smoke even more. However, the sensation of cooling the smoke is lovely. If you love bongs or water pipes, be sure to vape or use edibles sometimes too.

- Be careful with tobacco. Even with organic varieties, a number of carcinogenic compounds are produced in combustion. There are other smoking herbs and blends out there that can be added to change the strength and effect of the cannabis if you're interested in diluting it, though of course burning anything will mean inhalation of combusted matter.

> "You can look at the harm caused by free radicals as 'biological rust,' and the endocannabinoid system minimizes the impact of that and directly acts as an antioxidant."
> —Dr. Robert Melamede, professor of biology, University of Colorado Springs

VAPING

Vaping is the process of inhaling cannabis vapor. You can either vaporize ground cannabis flower or use a portable vape and concentrated cannabis oil.

PROS	CONS
In vaping the healing oils are essentially steamed from the plant matter, so your lungs are protected from the particles caused by combustion.	Because vaping can feel so mild compared to smoking, some people don't realize how much they're consuming until they're over the edge. Stoners call this the "creeper effect." Beginners should still go slow.
Vaping produces a cleaner, clearer terpene taste than smoking, so you can really appreciate the unique flavors of each strain instead of burning them off.	Many vape pen companies add a compound called propylene glycol (PG), which thins the cannabis oil so it flows through the pen better. Although said to be safe for food consumption (which is weird because it comes from petroleum), high temperatures break this substance down into polymers, which damage lung tissue, and carbonyls, which are a group of cancer-causing chemicals that includes formaldehyde! Adding insult to injury, many vape pens get so hot that the cannabis oil is in fact *smoldering,* bringing higher levels of damage from the PG.
Vaping is convenient and discreet, with a far less obvious smell, for those yogis who would prefer to be more subtle about enhancing.	
Many people find vaping provides an experience that has more of a "body" feel than smoking, which can be extra useful for yoga.	
Vaping tends to have a slower, more gradual onset, so that there is less of a jarring, "suddenly I'm high" feeling. This is great for beginners.	
I find vapes also provide a much milder effect than smoking, which is also good for beginners.	Vapes for cannabis flower, or ones where you add oil yourself, mitigate the need for petroleum products in our medicine, but many also damage terpenes from being too hot.

Tips

- Do some research and buy a vape pen that doesn't contain propylene glycol. Look for vegetable glycerin instead, if anything. E-mail your favorite pen company to see their white papers before purchasing. If they don't respond or if a pen doesn't have a lot of information online or on the packaging, skip it.

- Use a pen with a ceramic heating coil, so the propylene glycol doesn't get hot enough to release nanoparticles.

- Or make your own oil for self-fill cartridges by finding recipes online that mix hash with vegetable glycerin. New vapes have special attachments for oil concentrates.

- Buy vapes from a reputable company, as cheap construction may have dangerous metals or other chemical components. Avoid anything with an off smell; and to be safe avoid plastic or metal alloys altogether and just vapes made of food-grade glass or metal. (Food-grade plastic is better than nothing.)

GRINDER TIPS

1. Use a grinder to bust your bud, or else you'll waste delicious terpenes on your hands!

2. Use a grinder with a screen that catches the kief, which you can later sprinkle on joints or in pipes.

3. Take a nice whiff of your freshly ground bud before consuming it.

4. Don't overgrind your weed. Powdery ganja results in a loss of flavor and a harsher burn. Undergrinding, on the other hand, results in uneven burning and waste.

5. Clean your grinder regularly, so it doesn't gunk up and break.

- Use a convection vaporizer, instead of a conduction one, which ensures the heating element never touches the cannabis and you get the most complete terpene profile. Convection also provides more even heat distribution, so there's no need to stir the cannabis.

- The best temperature to vape cannabis flower is still argued about in stoner circles the world over. It's said to be between 157 and 210 degrees Celsius (314–410 degrees Fahrenheit).

- Although you expect not to, coughing from vaping happens, and it's a different kind of cough than from smoking. Don't feel self-conscious; just let yourself cough.

EDIBLES

Edibles are any cannabis taken as food. It may be a medicated olive oil you drizzle on salads, CBD lozenges, artisanal paleo protein bites, or the classic pot brownie.

PROS	CONS
Edibles are great for yoga, because they bring on an exquisite body high.	It may take up to ninety minutes to feel something, so if you want to be high when your yoga practice starts, you'll need to chow down quite a while before.
They're pragmatic, able to be added to any type of food or drink you can imagine.	This long onset can lead to overdose ("I don't feel anything yet!").
The onset for edibles is quite long, so some yogis like starting the practice while sober and allowing the high to slowly come in as the practice warms up.	Edibles can make it hard to do anything but the Corpse Pose. This is because THC is converted into a stronger form when it is absorbed by the liver instead of through the lungs.

Tips

- Start small, unless you want to practice "couchlock pose" all night.

- Be sure the edible is tested to confirm dosing.

- A good place for beginners to start is 5–15 milligrams of THC, if using. Those more experienced could try 15–30 milligrams. Wait two hours before adding more. Try 2:1 or 1:1 CBD/THC for more wellness, less trippy.

- Buy products that contain high-quality, whole-food, medicinal ingredients and go for low-glycemic sweeteners like maple syrup or agave.

- Look for edibles that contain coconut oil; it's high in saturated fat and can extract more cannabis than butter or other oils.

- To increase potency and enjoy a faster onset, consume the edibles along with nonmedicated food. More surface area of the stomach gets activated that way, meaning more acid to digest the weed.

- Store edibles in a cool dry place, in a container other than the plastic they may have been packaged in, to avoid petroleum-based estrogens from the BPAs.

TINCTURES

Tinctures are cannabis extractions (concentrates) that work sublingually, absorbed by the veins under the tongue (unlike edibles, which are absorbed through the stomach and liver).

For most of our country's history, cannabis was legal, commonly found in tinctures and extracts. Throughout the nineteenth century, American and European doctors prescribed cannabis tinctures to both children and adults for a variety of ailments from skinned knees to menstrual cramps.

PROS	CONS
Because they enter the bloodstream faster, tinctures work faster than edibles.	Decidedly the least fun method of consumption, tinctures are more medicinal than recreational.
The faster time makes them easier to dose than edibles. Instead of waiting two hours to see if you should add more, you'll know in twenty or thirty minutes.	

Tips

- Tinctures are normally made with alcohol or glycerin, and there is debate about which one is stronger and better for you. In any case, source a cold-extraction tincture if possible.

- To use a glycerin tincture, simply put a few drops under the tongue for twenty seconds to a minute before swallowing. You can make your tincture more effective by using your tongue to rub it on your inner cheeks as well. It's also been suggested that ten slow breaths in through the mouth and out through the nose make tinctures work better.

- If you're using an alcohol tincture, add it to a beverage.

- Store tinctures in a cool, dry place away from sunlight.

MICRODOSING

Microdosing is a new trend in cannabis wellness in which users find what's called the "minimum effective dose" to feel enhanced or even take doses too small to feel as a sort of homeopathic approach. It has been shown that even small doses of cannabinoids can have positive effects on neuropathic pain. Low doses of cannabis signal the body to both produce more endocannabinoids and build more cannabinoid receptors.

Many of us took part in a binge-smoking culture in high school and college. The ability to finally use something once prohibited led to heavy smoking. But with today's high test strains of cannabis, you can go incredibly far with just a puff or two.

Explore microdosing, small dosing, regular dosing, and megadosing to see how each affects your yoga practice and your life. Daily users who are not treating a specific condition should be very careful with megadosing, if for no other reasons than it is hard on the pocketbook and it is likely that you can get a similar response from a lower dose. Sometimes it feels good to get stoney baloney, and other times just a hoot will do it!

TOPICALS

Topicals are absorbed through the skin, activating the endocannabinoid receptors there. They're nonpsychoactive, but provide on-site relief of skin conditions and pain. Topicals come in an array of types, from lotions to bath salts, and they're often mixed with other healing herbs to help reduce muscle stiffness and tension.

PROS	CONS
Topicals are easy to use and are completely discreet. They are great for managing pain without changing your state of consciousness.	Anecdotally, I've heard many people say, "Most topicals don't work for me, but X does." That tells me that you may need to try a number of different topicals before you find one that works for you. In the worst case you will be rubbing a compound with strong antioxidants and hydrating oils into your skin.
Topicals lead to people administering self-massage more. Always a good thing!	

Tip

- Buy topicals that are made from food-grade ingredients. A good rule of thumb is not to put anything on your skin that you wouldn't put into your mouth.

RICK SIMPSON OIL

In 2003 Rick Simpson cured his skin cancer using a homemade cannabis remedy. Soaking cannabis in pure isopropyl alcohol causes the therapeutic compounds to be drawn out of the plant. After the solvent evaporates, the tar-like concentrate that remains is called RSO. Recipes online show you how to make this, or look for RSO in edibles or topicals.

CONCENTRATES

Dabbing is the name for ingesting concentrated cannabis compounds without combustion. A small amount of the concentrate is vaporized on a hot surface known as a nail; the vapor is then inhaled. Concentrates can also be sprinkled into joints or onto pipes, or used with certain vaporizers.

Methods of extracting the cannabis concentrates differ, as seen below, but they all strip the healing and psychoactive compounds from the plant resin, so the final product is much more heavily concentrated than the bud you put in your pipe. For instance, some concentrates are 80–90 percent THC, whereas cannabis flower is often only 18–22 percent. Other concentrates are made with cannabis flower that is rich in the nonpsychoactive but therapeutic cannabinoid CBD.

PROS	CONS
Dabbing is similar to the vape-pen experience. Concentrated cannabis oils are extraordinarily rich in cannabinoids and terpenes, making them very effective medicinals.	Some extraction methods use butane and other petroleum products, which cause nervous system disorders at high exposures.
The high is unique and powerful, but exquisitely clear and functional.	The whole dabbing process can be intimidating, as it involves a butane torch and some knowledge about when to apply the concentrate to the nail to maximize the effectiveness (although new products are coming on the market that use electric heat to replace the open flame).
	Dabs can be strong—strong and addictively good. I have friends who find joints too mild now.

THE FOUR MOST COMMON METHODS OF CONCENTRATE EXTRACTION

SOLVENT EXTRACTION

The most common type of concentrate is made with the use of solvents such as butane. The most important consideration for those who prioritize health is whether any residual solvent remains on the final product. If a toxic solvent like butane is not properly purged, we will be consuming it when we dab. A health-conscious option is to avoid butane-extracted concentrates altogether, especially if lab results showing residual solvents are unavailable.

CARBON DIOXIDE EXTRACTION

Concentrates extracted with carbon dioxide (CO_2) do not contain chemical solvents. CO_2 extraction uses pressure and carbon dioxide to separate plant material. This method is one of the safest and most effective ways of reducing cannabis to its essential compounds and leaves a product with a much higher terpene content than butane extraction. However, these concentrates tend to be more expensive than butane-extracted concentrates, and some methods remove and reintroduce terpenes, potentially changing the flavor and health effects.

ICE WATER EXTRACTION

Another solventless option is water-hash concentrates, which are also called bubble hash or full-melt hash. This is one of the safest and cleanest extraction methods and does not change the terpene profile. Testing has shown THC levels to be lower than CO_2- and butane-extracted oils, however, at potencies this high, the average yogi probably can't tell the difference. In this method, plant material is mixed with cold water and ice and then agitated to break off the trichomes (the little crystal hairs you can see on the cannabis flower that contain all the yummy cannabinoids and terpenes). The product is then filtered, leaving behind a pure final product that typically tests between 50 and 80 percent THC.

THE MAKING OF ROSIN

The newest type of extract on the scene right now, and the one most popular among health-conscious yogis, is rosin. This type of concentrate is not derived by the addition of any foreign substances, but rather is formed by a mechanical process involving heat and pressure. You can make rosin yourself in about fifteen seconds with a standard hair straightener, parchment paper, and some hand-applied pressure or a cheap clamp. When the cannabis flower is pressed and heated quickly between the parchment sheets, it extrudes the cannabinoids and terpenes, creating an oil that is similar in flavor and potency to that of high-quality water hash.

Tips

- Various concentrates have different consistencies and colors, each the result of a specific extraction process. Contrary to popular belief, appearance is not necessarily an indicator of quality. Only testing done by an analytic lab can ensure terpenes and cannabinoid contents.

- Avoid butane hash oil (BHO), the concentrate made by the butane extraction method. Even if the butane was "purged properly," there are alternatives on the market (see below), so we might as well avoid toxic chemical solvents if at all possible.

- It is essential that any concentrate be made from cannabis flower that was grown organically (without pesticides), for any impurities will be present—and concentrated—in the final product.

- Buy a quality, American-made quartz nail to dab from.

- Did I mention dabs are superstrong? First-timers should be in a comfortable space (internal and environmental), with plenty of water handy, and someone to take care of them if they're nervous. Ask an experienced friend to walk you through it, if possible. Take your first few dabs sitting down, just in case.

- Consider your strain and terpene profile, as you will definitely get more of the terpene effect from dabbing.

- Start small, half the size of a grain of rice. You can always add more.

- Don't hold your dab in, just take a full inhalation and then exhale.

If your hash is too firm to crumble up for a joint or pipe, stick it onto a pin and then warm it gently with a lighter until soft, being careful not to burn it.

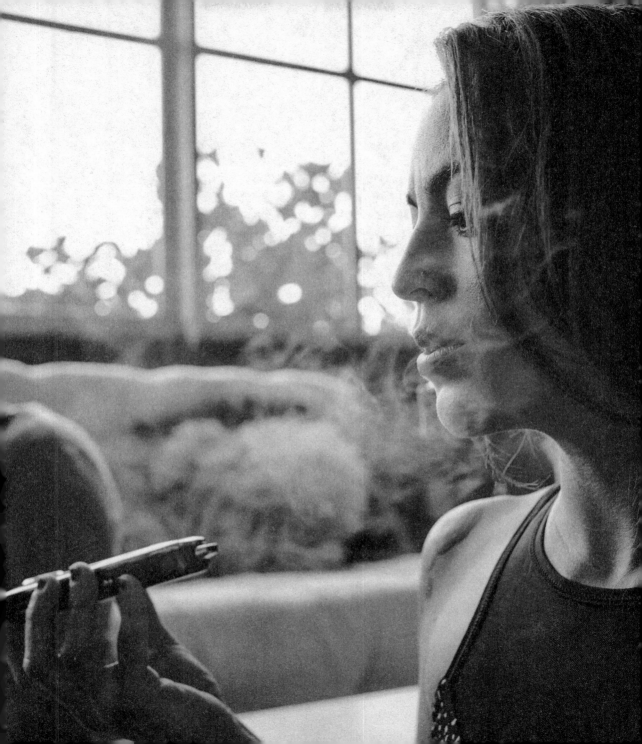

TEACH ME HOW TO DAB!

Okay, now you have the lowdown on concentrates. Time to dab. Using a blowtorch to get high may seem daunting at first, but pretty soon you'll get the hang of it and feel glad you stepped through the door into the most tasty, clean, instant, and healthy high on the market! (You can also check out my Ganja Yoga YouTube channel for an instructional video.)

WHAT YOU'LL NEED

- A propane or butane torch. The former gets hotter faster and is more affordable, but can be more difficult for beginners to manage.

- A "dab rig" (a specific type of water pipe designed for dabbing).

- A dab nail, which is a quartz, titanium, or ceramic piece that fits on the dab rig. Avoid glass, as it is less able to withstand high heat and could break. Some nails look like the head of a nail and come with a separate glass dome, whereas others are dome-shaped themselves.

- A metal "dab tool" to pick the sticky concentrate up with. (You could try an opened paper clip in a pinch.)

- A glass "carb cap" (the container your concentrates came in or a shot glass), to cover the nail as you consume, leading to a bigger, fuller hit.

- Somewhere comfy to sit, with a glass of water nearby.

- An attitude of relaxed openness.

- If you feel the need, an experienced dabber to accompany you on your initial foray.

STEPS

1. Make sure you have your gear all ready.

2. Turn on your torch and aim the flame directly at the nail, heating it until it gets red-hot, to fully clean off any old dab and ensure the cleanest taste. If your nail is dome-shaped, heat the bottom of the back end. Once the nail is hot, turn off your torch and place the glass dome over the nail (if your rig comes with one) and let the nail cool down. It's recommended to let titanium nails cool for about ten seconds and quartz nails about forty-five seconds, so the surface temperature isn't scalding hot. If you have a laser thermometer, make sure the temperature of the surface is between 350 and 440 degrees Fahrenheit; or you could hold your inner wrist just above it and gauge the temperature from that. The higher end of the spectrum causes a more thorough vaporization (more high), and the lower end of the spectrum preserves more delicious and healing terpenes.

3. Once your nail is cool, sit up tall with the chest open so you'll be able to breathe fully. Using your tool, apply the dab directly on the nail inside the dome or to the back of the dome-shaped nail. Immediately begin to inhale the vapor, doing so very slowly, at the same time rotating the dabber tip on the nail to get all of the concentrate off. Then put your dab tool down and, while still inhaling, use a "carb cap" to build more vapor and a more complete experience. Once you've inhaled all you'd like, do not hold the vapor in. Just take a nice comfortable hit, exhale, and see how it lands for a minute or so before taking a second one. (You can carb your nail and take a second hit from the same dab without reheating the torch.)

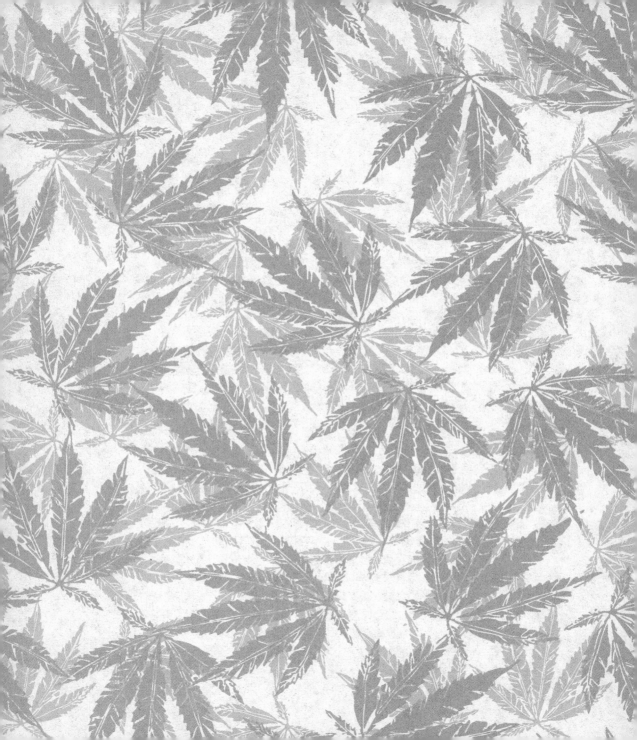

10

PURCHASING TIPS

MOST OF US KNOW THAT sativa-based strains are euphoric and uplifting, indica strains are calming, and hybrids are a bit of both, but with so many variables in cannabinoid and terpene content, simply dividing the plant into these three categories is far too simplistic. More progressive thinkers have taken a look at the impacts of terpenes and decided that the indica/sativa division is imaginary and in fact *unhelpful* in determining the experience you may have.

Traditionally it has been thought that sativa's tall stems and long, thin leaves meant it evolved in humid jungle climates, while indica's shorter stems and wider leaves meant it developed in more arid mountain and desert conditions. However, these claims are controversial, because both strains readily interbreed with each other, and both grow in diverse climates, with or without human assistance. As such, there is an increasing discussion among researchers about whether the existing classification is even accurate.

After examining decades of literature on the topic, cannabis researcher Dr. Ethan Russo recently stated in the journal *Cannabis and Cannabinoid Research* that he believes the sativa/indica distinction as we commonly use it is "total nonsense and an exercise in futility. One cannot in any way currently guess the biochemical content of a given cannabis plant based on its height, branching, or leaf morphology . . . because of the degree of interbreeding/hybridization." In other words, it's the ratio of THC to CBD and the terpenes present that determine what the experience will be like, not the shape of the leaf or the name.

Which Strain to Purchase?

So what is a ganja yogi to do? First, be sure your strain has some THC and some CBD as well as other cannabinoids, if possible, to ensure you're taking full advantage of the entourage effect.

The absolute best way to determine which strain to purchase is to stick your nose right into the big weed jar at the dispensary and notice which flavors (terpene combinations) you're most drawn to. First, stronger-smelling weed indicates that it is fresher and has more active terpenes. Second, cannabis that smells good to you might mean your body needs that particular form of healing. Health-conscious cannabis users do not go by the name or type of strain, but let the body's wisdom decide which cannabis strain is needed. Just as when you go to the farmer's market and decide what produce to purchase based on ripe smells, bright colors, or inexplicable cravings, let strain selection be an intuitive decision, based on your unique body chemistry and your body's ability to communicate with you (your mind).

This is important because each person has such an individualized relationship to cannabis, and there is such a vast range of cannabinoid and terpene constellations available. How a specific strain works on you will not be the same for your friend. Yogis are encouraged to start a weed journal, recording each strain tried, where it was purchased, what farm grew it (if available), and the cannabinoid content, if provided (sometimes only the amount of THC is given). As well, note any analytics provided for terpenes or purity, how you consumed it, and the kind and strength of high you felt. Download the log I created by visiting www.theganjayoga.com.

And for people thinking, "Just tell me a strain, and I'll do the smelling and journaling later," here you go. Sativa tends to offer a cerebral high, great for mood elevation and cognitive enhancement. Indica is more

For new users, it's best to find a dispensary you feel comfortable in, one that provides answers to your questions and lets you take as long as you need to make decisions. Delivery is cool, but there is simply nothing like working with an experienced and knowledgeable budtender. Choose delivery services that offer in-home consultations with their product.

sedative. A good place to start are hybrids, which offer a balance between the energizing effects of sativa strains and the relaxing effects of indica strains.

Yogic Buying Practices

Cannabis legalization and normalization in some states have given many of us a cornucopia of pot products to choose from. As the industry gains momentum, more and more amazing brands are popping up that prioritize health and wellness—for the consumers, the farmers, and the planet!

Ganja yogis share many of the same values, and these are the values we must vote for when we shop. As more companies compete for your dollar, to the best of your ability, make sure they follow some of these good-karma guidelines.

RESPONSIBLY FARMED

Plants grown in the sun are the most natural and sustainable. Indoor-grown plants get artificial light for three months. Outdoor cannabis plants get charged with the full spectrum of sunlight for a full eight months. This natural light spectrum produces more cannabinoids and terpenes (contrary to popular belief!), without the intensive resources indoor monocultures require for lighting, ventilation, cooling, and dehumidifying. Sun-grown cannabis also requires far fewer pesticides and fungicides, the residues of which can be extremely hazardous to your health.

Make sure you are purchasing cannabis from a farm that has tested the soil to see that it is free of heavy metal contamination. Cannabis is an excellent phytoremediator, meaning it soaks up all of the heavy metals in its immediate environment. Indeed, cannabis can even clean radioactive metals from soil. It is of paramount importance to your health that you source your cannabis from a responsible grower who is taking care to eliminate your exposure to heavy metals in your bud.

The exception to this is for medical users with compromised immune systems or other serious conditions who may have low tolerance for the natural variability of sun-grown, soil-grown plants. If this sounds like you, consult a doctor and a knowledgeable budtender.

ORGANIC, LOCALLY GROWN

Industrial fertilizers and chemical pesticides sprayed onto crops to increase yields are considered safe enough to eat, but when the same chemicals are smoked, they enter the bloodstream without being metabolized by the digestive tract. In addition, because of the disastrous federal prohibition of marijuana the FDA cannot regulate the industry. This means a nonorganic joint may have more neurotoxicity than a nonorganic apple! Worst of all, because the FDA is not involved, producers cannot legally label their products "organic."

When you specifically purchase products that are free of chemical fertilizers and poisonous pesticides, you show businesses that you want your medicine to remain all-natural. Plus it tastes better, because it was grown the way Mother Nature intended, and doesn't hurt the surrounding ecosystems. Look for a certification of organic from Clean Green, Certified Kind, or another third-party organization to ensure a cleaner, greener, more sustainable industry. At the very least, find a dispensary or producer that is clear and transparent with its testing process.

MEDICINAL INGREDIENTS

In your choice of edibles you should treat food as medicine, especially if you eat edibles often. Treats and indulgences are fine, but a whole-foods diet is what brings health, happiness, and longevity. Look for products that are free from processed ingredients, refined sugars, artificial preservatives, artificial sweeteners, trans fats, and food coloring. Buy organic if you can. If quality edibles don't exist where you live, create your own whole-food edibles with maple syrup or other healthier sugar alternatives.

TESTED FOR CONTAMINANTS, CANNABINOIDS, AND TERPENES

Good companies pay independent third parties to lab-test and certify their products are free from pesticides, molds from improper drying, and pathogens from improper extraction.

Cool weed companies let you know exactly how much of each type of medicine you're getting. Look for percentages of cannabinoids and terpenes on the website or labeled right on the package.

CORPORATE RESPONSIBILITY

Does your company donate a portion of sales to help bring an end to cannabis prohibition? Does it have a compassion program for low-income patients? Is its social media presence about lobbying for safe, affordable access for all people or does it only seem concerned with the bottom line? Does its marketing strategy consist of more tired images of women as objects of desire, or do its campaigns represent a variety of cannabis users?

FAIRLY FARMED, SMALL BUSINESSES

Buy from mom-and-pop shops, growers, and manufacturers who risked their livelihoods to end prohibition. In many cases, these people went to jail so you and I can legally smoke. As cannabis becomes legalized, Big Pharma, Big Alcohol, Big Tobacco, and corporations like Monsanto all have eyes on the profits to be made. Don't let factory farms dominate the market; keep this industry as compassionate, inclusive, and progressive as the people who created it, putting your hard-earned money into the hands of small, locally owned, community-minded businesses that care for patients. Do this because cannabis is not just another "consumer product." It's not a vice or an indulgence; it's a medicine for living healthier, more balanced, more meaningful lives and should be available to everyone.

WEED STORAGE AND HANDLING TIPS

Temperature, light, air, and time can all degrade terpenes and the strength of your medicine. Store ganja in a cool, dark, dry place in any container except plastic. Avoid touching cannabis flower with your hands, so you don't knock off your terps. Use chopsticks or a light touch to get your bud from the jar to the grinder, and then a folded card or spoon to get it from the grinder to a pipe or doobie.

Purchasing CBD Products

- CBD is often labeled by ratio, the stated amount of CBD relative to the stated amount of THC. A 1:1 ratio, where both of the two most prevalent cannabinoids are equally present, is a great place to start. The cannabinoids work synergistically at this level to bring the best pain relief.

- Anxiety relief can be felt at 2:1, though for a stronger effect try higher ratios, from 8:1 or up to 20:1. Antiseizure treatment needs far less THC than this, something like 30:1.

- CBD can also be labeled by total CBD percentage. Anything higher than 4 percent is considered high. Talk with your medical marijuana doctor and budtender, and do some research online to help you find the best formula for you.

- Try four or five different CBD products even if the first few don't work for you. The unique constellation of cannabinoids and terpenes in each individual strain, the different growing conditions between the same strains, and the unique physical composition of your body—all these variables mean a lot of experimentation may be required to find the perfect ratio and product.

- Hemp-derived CBD may contain toxic contaminants. This is because industrial hemp is a phytoaccumulator, meaning it absorbs the contents of its environment, including things like heavy metals from the soil. In some places, hemp-derived CBD is all that's legal right now, and for patients with great need, it's still better than nothing! If possible, make sure your provider sources hemp from clean soils, and grows organically.

- Although cannabinoids can be extracted from the rest of the plant, whole-plant medicine is more effective due to the entourage effect. Buy CBD products or flower that consist of *a blend of strains*, not just pure CBD extract.

- Keep in mind that CBD does not produce any psychoactive effects even at high ratios. However, experiencing a mind free of anxiety can feel so unusual that you might feel high.

Other Cannabinoids

Research is only just beginning on the lesser-known cannabinoids, but they're already showing further therapeutic effects. Cannabinol (CBN) is a result of oxidation of THC. It is far less psychoactive than THC, but brings about a strong sedative effect, which can be a desired outcome, though not when it's a surprise. Prevent your THC from turning to CBN by making sure it's not exposed to light, heat, or air for a prolonged period, and don't cook your edibles at too high a temperature or for too long. Unless of course you're using cannabis to fight insomnia or seizures, in which case, CBN is an exceptional remedy.

Cannabichromene (CBC), another nonpsychoactive compound of cannabis, provides sedative, anti-anxiety, and antidepressant effects while also stimulating brain growth. It has also been shown to enhance the pain-relieving potential of THC. Cannabigerol (CBG) has pain-relieving and anti-inflammatory properties, inhibits GABA uptake in the brain, leading to relaxation and reduced anxiety, and can reduce intraocular pressure for those with glaucoma. As the other seventy-five cannabinoids get researched, your whole medicine cabinet may be replaced!

Both cannabis and yoga will reduce pain, but without an anti-inflammatory diet (high in vegetables and low in sugar and starches) results may be limited.

Hemp and Hemp Seeds

Hemp is a nonpsychoactive strain of cannabis (low THC) bred to be used for food or industrial products like rope. Hemp can be used to help solve many of our environmental problems. For example, it can be used to make paper instead of chopping down rain forests, to make clothing instead of growing cotton (a crop that needs pesticides), and as biodiesel.

Hemp seeds are an extremely healthy food, offering benefits that few other foods provide. Like meat, hemp seeds are a complete protein, containing all twenty amino acids including the nine essential amino acids that the body cannot produce on its own.

Hemp seeds are very high in essential omega-3 fatty acids, building blocks required for healthy neurological functioning, mood regulation, and hormone production. Omega-3s also reduce the inflammation that leads to pain, heart disease, and cancer. Hemp seeds are also uniquely high in a type of omega-6 fatty acid called gamma linolenic acid. This essential compound further reduces inflammation, preventing a variety of health ailments. Hemp seeds are also high in vitamin E, an antioxidant, and many other minerals, as well as soluble and insoluble fiber, both of which are needed for good digestive health. They have been shown to stabilize appetite and strengthen the immune system.

Anandamide is the name of the molecule your brain makes that works on the same receptor site as the cannabinoid THC. Researchers named it after the Sanskrit word for "bliss" because of its spiritual, joy-giving effects.

Hemp seeds are like CBD; they do not change the state of consciousness other than providing a sense of well-being. In his last six years of asceticism before enlightenment, the Buddha is said to have subsisted on one hemp seed daily.

Tips

- Just as in buying flower or concentrate, make certain your hemp seeds come from plants grown in clean soils, free from heavy metals and toxins.

- Buy hulled hemp seeds and add them to smoothies, oatmeal, casseroles, or soups, or drizzle hemp-seed oil over salads or soups or into smoothies.

- Bonus: Need to buy a yoga mat? Be sure to purchase one made of hemp! Your mat-carrying bag can also be made from the sustainable plant.

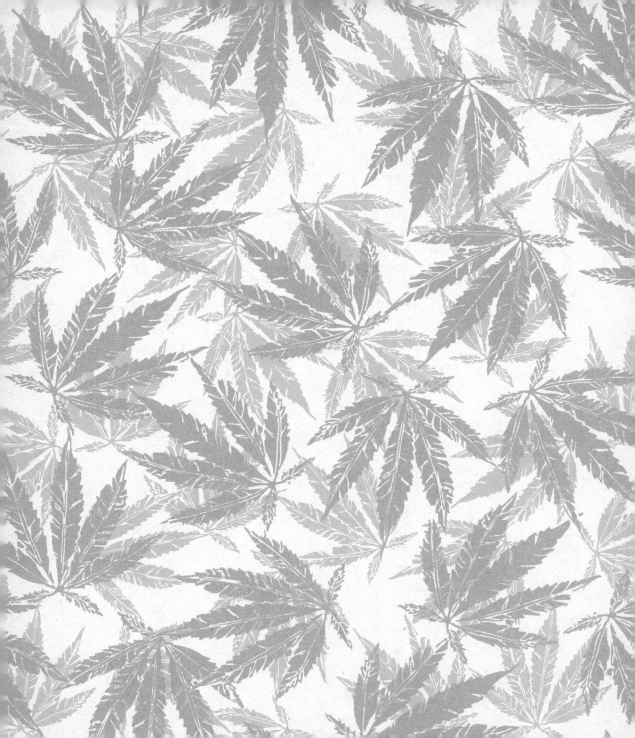

11

ENHANCING:
When, Where, and How Much

WE'RE ALMOST THERE, FOLKS. We know why weed is good for us. We've learned how it's been used spiritually by yogis. We know why the various practices of yoga—movement, stretching, breathing, mindfulness, and meditation—are beneficial for our bodies, minds, and spirits, and we also know how yoga and cannabis work together to safely and effectively produce the altered states of consciousness that have been called "spiritual experiences" by people all over the world throughout time. We also know the best practices to keep Ganja Yoga

123

safe, inside and out. We even know the types of cannabis products out there, and how to purchase the safest, most effective medicine that is also respectful of the planet. We are Ganja Yoga geniuses!

But before we blaze and bend, we need to be aware of the unique facets that will impact the actual yoga experience. These are called *setting* and *set,* and they change all the time.

Setting

Remember when we talked about intention? Intention plants the seed for your practice, while setting and set are the ways in which that seed comes into fruition, the concrete circumstances that will affect the environment and experience. Remember your personal intentions and rituals as we explore the practical parts of Ganja Yoga—the *when, where,* and *how much.*

One of the most important factors when getting high for yoga, or really anytime you're going to smoke, is to ensure that the *setting,* the environment, is conducive to a relaxing experience. Consider the things that affect your nervous system's ability to relax: lighting, music, other noise, warmth, privacy, having enough space to move, the energy of others, and so forth.

Your clothing is a part of this; make sure you wear something in which you can breathe comfortably and move around fully. Choose textures that are soft and pleasing. Awareness practices increase our sensitivity, so that we may discover stressors we hadn't considered before. The more we become aware of stressors (like synthetic fabrics that don't "breathe"), the more we can eliminate them, so we are starting from a higher baseline of bliss in our toke-yoga sessions.

GANJA YOGA PLAYLIST

Music makes the mood, and there are a number of different moods to choose from for your enhanced yoga on any given day. Folksy? Trippy? Soulful? Here are my top ten songs for Ganja Yoga. Check out all my playlists at www.theganjayoga.com!

1. "Natural Mystic," by Bob Marley
2. "Ghostwriter," by RJD2
3. "Crystal Rope," by Gayngs
4. "Samidha's Tune," by Harry Manx
5. "My Sweet Lord," by George Harrison
6. "It Is So Nice to Get Stoned," by Ted Lucas
7. "Krishna Dub Remix," by MC Yogi
8. "Angels," by The xx
9. "Hej, Me I'm Light," by Phosphorescent
10. "Shamanic Dream," by Anugama

Set

Set is your *mind-set,* your mood and energy level, and your *intention* for the practice. Some things that affect your mind-set are your health, how recently you ate, your diet in general, what kind of sleep you've had recently, and the kind of day you're having.

Some things related to your intention are the method of cannabis ingestion (a topical, tincture, vape, joint, bong hit, and fat dab all do very different things, all else considered) and dose, quality, and strain (available cannabinoids and terpenes). Once more, mindfulness training helps us to be better at checking in with ourselves, so we can choose cannabis strains, yoga practices, and types of music that are in alignment with our intention for the practice.

Don't consume if it doesn't feel right, even if you don't know why it doesn't feel right. Be mindful and trust your intuition. Reservations felt before lighting up can become magnified under the lens of cannabis. There will always be another opportunity to get high. The more you listen to your inner voice, the better your intuition will serve you.

Where to Do Cannabis-Enhanced Yoga

Where you practice Ganja Yoga depends on what's available to you and what you prefer. You could:

- Go to a cannabis-enhanced yoga class if there's one in your city.
- Go to a regular yoga class while high.
- Get high at home with friends and do yoga.
- Do Ganja Yoga alone.

Let's visit each scenario.

GOING TO A CANNABIS-ENHANCED YOGA CLASS

The whole is greater than the sum of its parts. At Ganja Yoga classes you get to consciously use cannabis to quiet the mind, relax the body, and tap into yourself alongside others who are doing the same.

Teachers and classmates know you're blazed, so you don't have to get paranoid and try to hide it. Each enhanced class will be totally different, depending on the teacher's style of yoga and presentation of the pairing, the strains and methods used, and the unique personalities who show up to class.

Tips

- Read the promotional material in print or online so you know what to expect, and arrive in plenty of time for your first class, so you're not rushed and out of sync with your body.

- You may want to develop a relationship to cannabis before attending a Ganja Yoga class. Although not required (for indeed my classes are a relaxing, safe space for first-timers), you might find your experience in a group setting to be more enhanced if you survey the stoner landscape at home a few times first.

- Bring along a friend if you feel nervous. That way you'll have a familiar face to turn to when the walls start melting (ha-ha, just kidding). If you go alone, make a point of introducing yourself to some classmates, and if there are any regulars, ask what keeps bringing them back to class. Knowing what others liked about the experiences might calm any nerves you have.

- Don't feel pressured to consume as much (or as little) cannabis as your classmates.

- Don't be nervous about "secret" stoner "rules of conduct," like which way you should pass the joint. Usually it's to the left, but it doesn't really matter. People's rules and etiquette preferences vary, but if you are all there for yoga, you're there to *shed worry and anxiety,* not create more of it. Generally don't bogart (hog), and you'll do okay. Remember, the joint is not a microphone.

- As practice begins, close your eyes and tap into your body, regardless of what's going on with the class. As long as you're not harshing other people's buzz, you have the freedom to do whatever it takes to relax, like yawning or sighing to get more in touch with your body.

- Bring water in case it isn't provided, and a protein-rich snack to munch on afterward.

GOING TO A REGULAR YOGA CLASS WHILE HIGH

Going to a regular (sober) yoga class while secretly stoned is sneaky fun. Although I share my story (on the next page) of consuming a buttload of cannabis before an Ashtanga class because it was funny, I actually *don't recommend taking extreme doses in situations where everyone else is sober,* unless you are very familiar with that type of yoga practice, that teacher, and that studio, and have a friend to be your partner in crime if things get hairy. Wavelengths that different could lead to conflict or anxiety, and flow-based classes that move quickly could cause you to injure yourself. Having shared my story, I offer some more tips for doing it right.

Tips

- Dose small. You can always add more, but you can never add less.

- Have some proficiency with cannabis and with being high around other people who aren't high to ensure you'll be relaxed if you attend sober yoga class while high. Even better, have a basic proficiency in yoga as well.

- Edibles in particular can knock you on your ass, so experiment at home.

UNDERCOVER GANJA YOGA

Earlier that morning, Stuart showed up with fresh, unpasteurized (illegal) cow's milk, sacred nectar to any Hindu. We had our organic cannabis, which wasn't easy to find in Ontario, and we had our rose water, cardamom, and ghee. We carefully stirred the milkshake 108 times while chanting incantations to Shiva, and after imbibing an enormous dose of the sacred elixir, we set out to a sober yoga class.

A total weed lightweight at the time, by registration I could already feel my eyeballs rolling around in my head. I signed the waiver and stumbled into the packed studio ready to secretly unite with Shiva while my classmates simply worked on their Scorpion. . . .

My body is moving through the Ashtanga Flow Sequence because I have it memorized, but I've never been this baked before, so my mind is all white walls and tiny rainbows. I hear the teacher's voice, and some reptilian part of me moves with it, Upward Dog, Lunge, Downward Dog, but I can't tell if my eyes are open or closed or what direction I'm facing. Sweat pours off me in this heated room; each drop tickles, and I want to giggle, but the rest of the class is serious, so I keep at it.

I think I'm keeping up with the group, but really I'm not thinking at all. There's no group, there's only me. Maybe it's easier. Stuart wasn't able to put his mat near mine in this packed class. I can't check in with him to see if he's also trapped in melting see-through sugar-ice like I am. But I ride the magic-carpet ride in this superchallenging practice (one that would have kicked my ass sober), until we all find Corpse Pose at the end. I am in the stillness of it, with ecstatic waves of energetic rainbow-bliss shooting out from my pelvis and filling my body with joy. I am one with Shiva.

- If the class is crowded, be aware the cannabis may make you dizzy and mess with your balance postures. Feel free to practice by a wall, just in case.

- You don't have to hide the fact that you're stoned, but you don't have to flaunt it.

- Bring along some water and a high-protein snack.

- New to yoga? Go to a beginner or restorative class or a class with the word "slow" in the title. Failing that, try a hatha class. Classes that offer more exercise—yoga like Vinyasa Flow, Ashtanga, Bikram, or anything with the word "power" in it—might not be suited to cannabis use, though that is my personal preference and opinion. *You do you*.

- Speaking of that, don't worry one bit what others are doing. The class you are at isn't designed for stoners. Rest when you need to and take care of you. Having said that, if you're becoming disruptive (if you're flailing all over in your balancing poses or laughing hysterically), quietly step out of the room to get your cool again, out of respect for the teacher, the practice, and your fellow students.

DOING GANJA YOGA AT HOME WITH FRIENDS

Sharing some nice bud with friends, shaking off the day, and connecting over a few laughs is the perfect way to start a yoga practice. Whether you all watch videos online, take turns leading, or do your own thing on the mat alongside each other, Ganja Yoga with friends is an awesome way to bring conscious relaxation into socializing. My husband and I got rid of our sofa and have yoga mats spread out instead, so we can arrange our bodies' joints into new positions as we hang with friends.

Tips

- Here you can customize your Ganja Yoga space with candles (placed safely!), your favorite music, and any objects that remind you to slow down, find meaning, feel good, and focus on what's important. Sometimes setting up an altar where everyone brings three objects that are meaningful or beautiful to them sets the tone for the consciousness to journey into more spiritual states.

- Everyone can use cannabis methods, strains, and doses that suit them, and it's never uncool to decline weed or say, "I've had enough."

- One person can be designated as leader for the session, to ensure the toking circle doesn't end up chatting all night. Decide beforehand if in the practice everyone will be taking turns presenting their favorite video on YouTube, leading their favorite meditation, or reading from a yoga book, or if you are all going to do your own thing to beautiful music until the timer goes off.

- Avoid "everybody look at me as I contort in this weird way" ego trips and, instead, focus on relaxing and tapping inward.

- As always, water and protein are nice to have handy.

TIPS FOR ANY GROUP YOGA CLASS

- **Never compare yourself to anyone else in the class.**

- **It's better to rest than to push.**

- **Close your eyes and feel.**

- **Other than the pleasure they bring you, your yoga mat or clothes don't matter.**

- **You have nothing to prove.**

SOCIAL STONER TIPS

- Cannabis users are a generous culture. Let's continue that as the industry builds. Share freely, accept gifts graciously, and don't get into the habit of mooching!

- Don't feel the need to consume the same amount or strain of weed as the people you're hanging with. We all have different relationships to the herb, and we've seen already that each strain will have its own terpene profile and effect on the body. I may need help with anxiety, while you may need help with lethargy. Don't harsh people's buzz by commenting on the fact that they smoke more or less than you.

- Pass to the left, usually. People who get rulesy aren't as fun to get high with.

- Make eye contact and smile when you pass, at least the first time.

- There's no shame in coughing, and those who tease their peers for coughing shall accrue seven additional rebirths in the endless cycle of life, suffering, death, and rebirth, according to Hindu mythology.*

- Don't bogart that joint, my friend.

  * Not a fact.

DOING GANJA YOGA ALONE

Doing yoga high can be most relaxing when you're all alone, because you can have everything to your own preference and not worry about other people's needs or expectations. After my husband goes to bed, I love lighting candles, playing Erykah Badu, and smoking some hash. Me time. Once a week or so, it's my witchy late-night yoga practice, where I spend hours in a dreamy state of consciousness that I can't always find time for during my busy days. Nothing beats loving your own company!

Tips

- Create the scene for relaxation before you get blazed. What could you do to enhance this relaxing experience, to create "nonordinary" space? Change the lighting? Play music you don't usually listen to? Definitely put your phone away. You might also set up an altar, which is a small table (or fabric on the floor) with objects placed on it that feel meaningful to you. You could also place sacred objects at the top of your mat to help you stay connected to your intention.

- Again, start with a small dose of weed; have water handy and a protein-rich snack for afterward.

- You can do spontaneous movements that feel good (yoga means "union," so as long as your mind, body, and awareness are all together, it's yoga!), or you can do videos online that are geared toward relaxation.

> If you are doing Ganja Yoga after work, taking a few minutes to blow off steam with a brisk walk or washing away the cares of the day in a shower can shake off some of the superficial layers of tension, so you are able to get into your stoner yoga session more quickly.

When to Get High for Yoga

Cannabis-enhanced spiritual practice has no direct lineage of texts (at least not translated into English) and thus has no masters, rules, or doctrines. When working with plant spirit medicines, shamans the world over acknowledge it's the spirit that resides in the plant itself that brings us inspiration.

As such, there is no suggested guideline for frequency, timing, or even dosing other than to be mindful as you consume. You might con-

TIPS FOR CANNABIS NEWBIES (and Everyone!)

- Set aside a big chunk of time for each of your first few cannabis experiences, so you can see what it's like without distraction or rush.

- Check in with your set and setting: make sure you're comfortable inside and out and have anything you might need at hand. It's normal to feel slightly nervous at first, but really tap inward to ensure the situation is right.

- Have an activity (like yoga!) planned. Most things you enjoy doing are even better high. If you're not sure what you might like to do, set out your yoga mat, some coloring books, and some massage cream and see where the afternoon takes you.

- Breathe and relax. Go with the flow. If anything feels weird about being high, lie down comfortably and know that everything passes. If you tend to get anxious, have a CBD tincture handy.

- Stay hydrated to avoid cottonmouth and have food handy in case you need it later.

- Don't worry if you don't feel anything the first time. With persistent effort you'll be flying high.

sume only before or do so throughout the practice. You might do yoga, then get high after as a reward.

Yoga poses can be mechanical when we lapse into inattentiveness, and likewise regular use of cannabis can become unconscious. Go slow. Take as much or as little weed as feels right. You can always add more, but you can never add less. Stay mindful.

Ganja Yoga Troubleshooting

Practicing preventative care is not as common as treatment of symptoms in our culture. Think of all the money, energy, and pain we all would save if we practiced prevention regularly, or if doctors got paid when you were healthy and feeling well instead of on a per-treatment basis. Yes, that would mean doing far more movements than we do now, eating far more vegetables, learning about herbs, supplements, and the basics of biology, nutrition, and biomechanics, and how to optimize our short time on earth . . . But wouldn't it be worth it?

Here are some ways to prevent common cannabis-related effects that can negatively impact your yoga practice. Most of them are useful for cannabis experiences off the mat too.

That said, sometimes things don't always go as planned, even with preventative self-care. For this reason I've also listed treatments for when something's already gone wrong.

In all cases, don't worry. Most of the time, the worst that may happen is that you forget what you were saying mid-sentence or you stretch the left hip twice. No biggie!

AGITATION AND ANXIETY

At the right strain and dose, cannabis removes excess noise from the mind. When there's too much THC, cannabis can create a mental whirlwind, leaving us overstimulated to the point of paranoia and panic.

Prevention

- If you don't like cannabis because you previously consumed too much and became anxious and withdrawn (like I used to), learn to fall back in love with the plant by experimenting with small doses in relaxing settings where you can control your surroundings. Over time, you'll learn to titrate (mindfully monitor) your dose, and can begin to add more or consume in less secure environments.

- Stick to lower-THC strains, as other cannabinoids mitigate the adverse effects of THC. Or try indicas, as they have terpenes that assist in bodily awareness and relaxation rather than energizing the mind.

- Add other smokable herbs to your joints or vapes. Damiana, mullein, catnip, and blue lotus are just some of the legal smokable herbs out there that you can add to decrease the potency of your ganja while still enjoying the experience.

- Interestingly, up to one in five people are not suited to THC because they lack the enzyme that breaks down anandamide (the naturally occurring endocannabinoid that resembles THC). As a result, these people have a higher baseline for it, and additional THC causes anxiety. If these prevention tips don't help, stick to higher-CBD strains, cannabis topicals, and hemp protein powder.

Treatment

- Citrus has been prescribed for supercharged tokers since the tenth-century Persian Empire! Recent studies have shown why: limonene has an extremely powerful anti-anxiety effect. Next time you get overcharged, sip some lemonade, preferably fresh squeezed and with pulp.

THAT'S DOPE

Cannabis causes the brain to releases a mild to moderate amount of the brain chemical dopamine, which is part of the reason it feels so good. However, it doesn't "flood the brain with it," as the media often reports.

The neurotransmitter dopamine is involved in many processes, though it's best known for its role in our seeking pleasure and reward, specifically with regard to addiction. However, dopamine is not a villain; it's a naturally occurring motivator. When levels go up, there is more desire to be productive and get things done. Although implicated in addiction to cocaine and amphetamines, in which less and less of the "feel good" dopamine rush happens as we get sensitized, dopamine works completely differently in the brain when THC or anandamide (our naturally occurring cannabinoid) is present.

- CBD tinctures are the safest, fastest-acting way to counterbalance anxiety induced by too much THC. Follow the instructions on the label and hold the tincture under your tongue for at least ten slow breaths. (Unless it's alcohol-based, in which case add to a beverage.)

- If possible, smooth out the rough edges of THC overdose with dim lighting, and do something relaxing and distracting, like coloring or watching kitten videos. Remember, as bad as it feels, in the long history of human cannabis consumption, there have been zero deaths as a result of overdose. Keep breathing and float downstream, knowing it won't last forever and that many, many of us (myself included) have been there!

- Stay hydrated, be sure you're warm enough, and baby yourself. This is a chance to feel compassion for your body. It's absolutely normal to feel unsteady, overwhelmed, and disoriented at first.

- Practice mindfulness. Look at the contents of your anxious mind. Journal or talk it out if that feels appropriate. Use this "bad trip" as a chance to look at your issues, a healing opportunity for personal growth.

- If you feel cannabis-induced paranoia during yoga, try Child's Pose. Kneel on your knees and lower legs, sit down on your heels, and bend forward till your forehead is on the mat or on a pillow. You can have your arms extended over your head or by your sides, and you can place a pillow under the belly or the bum for added comfort. Stay here and breathe slowly. The Child Pose is known by yogis to reduce sympathetic nervous system activation, reducing feelings of anxiety and being overwhelmed.

WORKING WITH SOCIAL ANXIETY

- If you're feeling a THC overdose in a public yoga class, take Child's Pose, quietly walk to the restroom to chill, or get some fresh air—alone or with a trusted friend.

- If you're getting high with friends, sometimes acknowledging to the group that you're feeling pot paranoia can make it go away or, at the very least, explain to others why you might be acting weird.

- If possible, take CBD in a fast-acting tincture and/or citrus to mitigate the uncomfortable effects of too much THC.

- Stay hydrated, breathe, and remember, this too shall pass.

LETHARGY AND LAZINESS

The media-created myth that cannabis causes laziness started as a racial stereotype of "lazy" Mexican workers and their "marijuana." (The racist heritage of prohibition is so pervasive and powerful that many activists refuse to use the word "marijuana," opting instead for the scientific term "cannabis.") For the most part, this stereotype goes on unquestioned in portrayals of cannabis users in the media today.

In contrast, many successful sports stars and Hollywood celebrities have admitted to smoking pot, along with countless intellectuals and artists. The "successful stoner" meme has exploded. Even President Obama inhaled. Clearly, then, cannabis does not lead to demotivation syndrome. In fact, Jamaicans use ganja to *aid* manual labor. However, some weed has terpenes and cannabinoids with sedative, tranquilizing effects, which is good weed for insomnia, catching up on sleep after a party weekend, or maybe even a restorative yoga class, but bad weed for getting off the couch when you're already late for your three o'clock Toke & Stretch date.

Prevention

- If you're always getting drowsy from cannabis, you might be smoking old weed, in which the THC has turned into the more sedating CBN. Or you're smoking a lot of indica with the terpene myrcene. CBD can also bring sleepiness. If you're treating insomnia, these give the desired effect, but for yoga we want some degree of motivation and alertness. Play around with strains, keeping a journal to note which ones give you more energy. Get recommendations from your budtender or doctor, and do some research online. Learning how your unique body responds to cannabis can become a fun adventure. Soon you'll find strains and doses that are effective but without the adverse effects.

Treatment

- If you wanted to do yoga and now after imbibing you're finding you're not in the mood, you could accept this new direction, let go of attachment to yoga, and relish in the new activity. If this whimsy feels right and there are no negative thoughts about having missed your practice, then it's a great choice. The other great choice when you don't feel like doing that thing you know you wanted to do before blazing is to "fake it till you make it." One. Foot. At. A. Time.

- It's normal to have yoga resistance even when you're sober. Every time I've felt too lazy to get to the studio and yet I forced myself to go, I've been reenergized and so glad I went. Just do it. Especially if you try the former choice but can't stop thinking about how you should go. Just go!

HOW TO REMOTIVATE YOURSELF

The right dose and strain will not demotivate you from enjoying the things you like. Getting on the floor and stretching, watching comedy, getting a massage, going for a hike, having a great conversation, and getting busy between the sheets all come more easily to me when I'm high. If you're finding you're too lazy or tired to enjoy even your favorite activities, bring mindfulness to that happening, and decide if you want to accept it ("I don't feel like yoga practice after all; I think I'd rather lie down and daydream"), or if you want to practice going against the gravity of lethargy ("Okay, I am very sluggish, but I can do just five minutes of stretching before bed"). If you decide to remotivate yourself, know that the first time is the hardest, the second is worlds easier, and the third, nothing at all. The brain is plastic, and you can change even deep neural grooves toward sluggishness and inertia.

DISTRACTION

"Salience" is a word that describes when things feel especially meaningful, prominent, or important. When we are mindful, more of life feels salient. Cannabis enhances salience, making yoga, sex, nature, music, philosophical debates, and even time with a doggie friend feel more special and meaningful.

For this reason, cannabis can actually cause you to work *harder* in meditation practice. Every thought is the best thought ever, but you are supposed to watch them and then let them go, not energize them.

I'm not here to say you *must* meditate when you want to jot down your incredible ideas! Just like you're the only one who can decide if you truly are best served lounging on the couch or overcoming lazy impulses, sometimes it feels right to go with the flow and let the creative muse inspire you. Other times, you want to concentrate on your yoga practice, and weed can be distracting.

Prevention

- Make this easy for yourself: no notebooks and pens near the yoga mat. (And definitely no cell phones!)
- Stick to lower THC strains to mitigate cognitive overload.

Treatment

- Surrender is a big part of yoga. Let those exceptional ideas go and return to your breath, trusting they'll come back later when you're able to record them. This cultivates more willpower. If ideas keep returning, keep returning to your yoga. That's why it's called a *practice*.

- Redirect your focus. Use the salience of cannabis to your advantage, helping you appreciate aspects of reality you may have missed. Once you do start to notice your breathing or the feeling of your body stretching in a posture, these sensory aspects of the present moment can become as fascinating as your most genius thought.

CLUMSINESS

At higher doses, cannabis may create a different kinesthetic connection with the body, including a slight decrease in coordination and reaction time. However, an extensive review of studies in a journal called *Accident Analysis and Prevention* found no statistically significant increase in car accidents as a result of cannabis use.

Experienced yoga practitioners might notice that the physical aspects of yoga can take some getting used to while under the influence. If you have a preexisting yoga practice with lots of precision, balance, or strength, you might find yourself wobbling in a pose for the first time in years or even clumsily falling out of it. Beginners to cannabis may even become dizzy. If this happens, slowly lower yourself to the floor and rest, eyes closed, until the spell passes. Rise again very slowly.

> Less is more. When teenagers smoke cannabis, they often try to show off how much they can consume (the way frat boys guzzle beer at parties). This level of intoxication, although fun at times, does not lend itself to a balanced wellness experience, whether you're relaxing on the beach, making love, hanging with friends, or doing yoga.

Prevention

- Use the yogic tool of self-awareness to monitor your high. Make a habit of asking yourself, "How are my cannabis levels?"

- Play with microdosing if you were so high last time that your body connection was severely hindered.

Treatment

- See this as a chance to laugh at yourself, to shed the ego-based notion of "perfecting," "attaining," or "accomplishing" postures; let the cannabis bring a mind-set in which you lose perfectionism and just *be*, regardless of what's happening with your body.

- Be compassionate in balancing poses. Cannabis can negatively impact that part of practice for some people. Use a wall for support, if needed, with as little contact between the hand and the wall as possible (e.g., three fingers, one, or just the pinkie), or just surrender and wobble, letting go of a need to be "perfect," because, honey, you already are.

LESS THAN MINDFUL CONSUMPTION

Clearly, cannabis can be used for pain relief, stress reduction, healing, and spiritual insight. On the other side of the coin, cannabis can be used to numb out from the challenges of reality. Which, if I may say, *is a totally healthy thing to do sometimes!*

You, me, each of us, we are *biological organisms*. Like all animals, we have bodies that are responsive, and the scary news stories, notifications, and environmental stressors of modern life naturally overwhelm the nervous system, which was not designed to deal with the relentless influx of stimulation.

Stress hurts! It's a natural response for an animal to want to get away from the situations and thought patterns that feel stressful. Whether your version is a vacation, hot bath, or hibernating in a cocoon of cannabis haze, putting down individual and planetary concerns for a little while, and tapping into something grander, is what yoga is all about.

It's good for us, as organisms, to not always have full consciousness of the suffering going on inside and around us. There's something to the "turn on and drop out" idea from the 1960s.

However, healthy escapism is one thing, and dependency is quite another. Cannabis is not physiologically addictive; your brain doesn't come to depend on cannabis for dopamine or GABA the way it does for cocaine and alcohol and other drugs that are typically abused. Having said that, everything that gives pleasure can cause dependency.

Dependency on cannabis exists when you continue to partake even though it causes you significant impairment or distress. Some of the consequences of cannabis dependence are decreased motivation toward participating in activities, failing to take care of obligations, social withdrawal, suspicion, and low agreeableness. Cannabis dependency is said to affect 9 percent of users, significantly less than alcohol and tobacco dependency at 15 percent and 32 percent.

Every molecule of the food, medicine, supplements, and drugs you consume will be processed by your body, and too much of any one thing, whether cannabis, coffee, water, or almond butter, isn't going to serve you long-term.

How much is too much? Cannabis is potentially the most vastly applicable healing medicine humanity knows of and a completely necessary medicine for many, many people. The purpose of this section is not to say regular or heavy cannabis use is not functional or appropriate; only *you* know how much is too much, only you know when your *use* becomes *abuse*.

Treatment and Prevention

- If your cannabis dependency causes significant impairment to your life or distress to you or your loved ones, the first step is to bring in awareness. Be mindful about your relationship to the plant and see if you can accept that there is an imbalance. You don't have to *do* anything about it right now.

- If you don't want to cut down, start to practice diversity in the types of cannabis you consume, so at least you're getting a variety of cannabinoids and terpenes. Try weaker strains earlier in the day when your tolerance is lower. Use a variety of consumption methods, especially if you dab a lot, and sometimes practice sobriety too for variety.

- Cannabis isn't the food itself; it's the spice that enhances life. If we use only one tool to offer ourselves stress relief, pleasure, and self-care without cultivating the sometimes effortful aspects of psychological development, we miss out on the full healing potential of the medicine. Try combining cannabis with art therapy, journaling, stress reduction, and other forms of self-discovery, relaxation, and personal growth. (Combining it with yoga is just the beginning!)

- Do a cannabis fast. Decide how long and stick to it, starting with a small, attainable goal. Will you fast for the morning today? Every morning this week until breakfast? The whole day? Three days? Three weeks? A good thing about a break, even a short one, is that you reset your tolerance and need less cannabis to feel the effect.

- Specific to yoga itself, practice without cannabis sometimes. Being sober highlights certain aspects of yoga that being high doesn't, like really getting in touch with the sense of boredom that can arise when there's always cannabis salience to delight us in familiar poses. Sometimes it's useful to practice being with boredom, since it's a state so many of us have become completely intolerant of in the cell-phone age.

Again, this is advice specifically for those who are *suffering* from their dependency. I know here in San Francisco, many successful people are lifted from the time they wake up, and they suffer none of these consequences. When they travel somewhere where cannabis isn't available, they don't have withdrawal, so they have no need to try and live without it. Other people have serious medical needs, cannabis is their primary treatment option, and they should not live without it. Everyone's body chemistry is different, so we all have a completely unique relationship to this complex healing herb. Only you know if you need to take a break.

> Just because things that bring pleasure may cause addiction doesn't mean we stop doing them— smelling flowers in the park, eating ice cream, or having hot sex with a new lover. Why would we be afraid of enhancing yoga with a safe substance that can bring the brain chemistry of bliss that our yogic forefathers described?

From the tantric perspective, there are no inherently right or wrong choices as long as we bring in awareness. Existence offers us so many gifts to help us awaken our consciousness, we would be foolish not to take advantage of them. If we're using the herb not to escape reality, but to experience it with fewer disturbances of the mind and gain more insight, the relationship is functional.

We will have our own rhythms and preferences for the frequency and dose of the cannabis we use, for yoga and for anytime, just as we have differences in how often we do yoga, what kind of yoga we do, the music we like for practice, whether we practice in the morning or evening, alone or with friends, on a sticky mat or pile of blankets, in a sexy sports bra, flannel pajamas, or naked. There is no right way to practice yoga. If it serves you, it is the "right way."

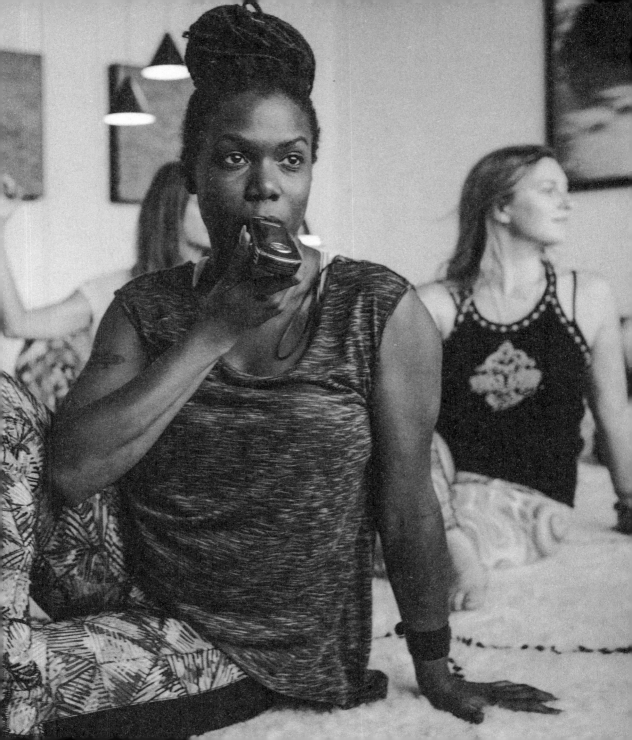

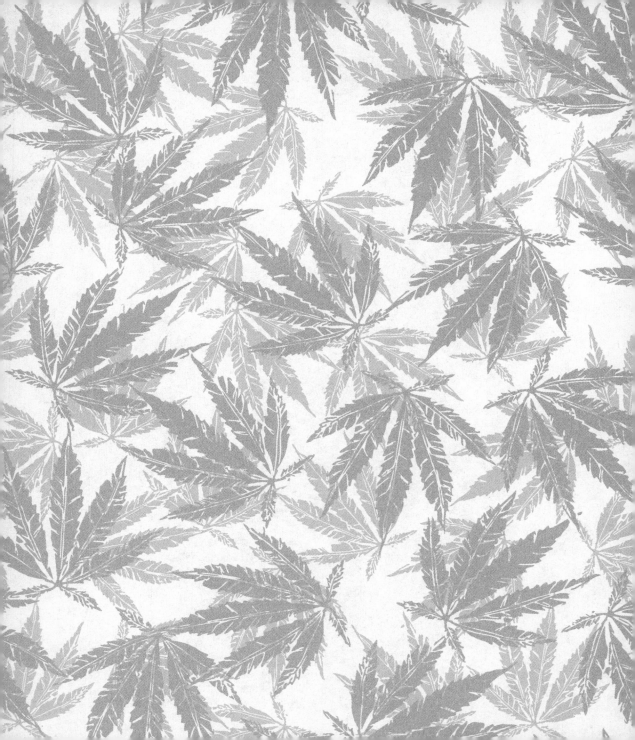

12

BAKED BREATHING PRACTICES

OUR CULTURE IS VERY VISUAL. Yoga magazine covers depict only the postural part of the practice not because postures are the essence of yoga, but because we can't easily show inner states of consciousness, breathing, and other subtle experiences in a way that sells magazines.

Postures may get all the attention, but like mindfulness *the breath is a more important part of yoga than the shapes or movements the body makes.* To do yoga postures without awareness of the breathing is to simply do calisthenics (which are still useful, but not necessarily yoga).

It is the breath that deepens the experience of being in a body. It takes us into poses, nourishes our tissues while we are in them, and lets us know when it's time to release.

A good yoga practice endeavors to keep the mind connected to the breath. We learn to bring the awareness back to the breath when it wanders, and we learn to link the breath to our movements, which helps us to truly feel the effects of each pose instead of zoning out.

Why We Need to Practice Deep Breathing

According to yoga, the way we breathe determines how much life-force energy we have. Breathing brings fresh air in and pushes waste air out. Inhalation happens when the diaphragm pulls down and reduces air pressure within the lungs relative to the outside air. As a result, air rushes into the lungs. If we're relaxed and our clothing is loose, the belly will softly rise on each in-breath and lower on each out-breath, the diaphragm moving like a bellows.

We are usually unconscious of our breath, and it's often shallow. Weak postural muscles, constricting clothing, sucking the belly in to appear slimmer, and trying not to experience unpleasant or inconvenient emotions all restrict deep breathing. In shallow breathing we're using mostly the upper chest muscles to open the rib cage. The image of an inflated chest and a flat belly might look sexy, but it only makes use of a fraction of your lung capacity. *Too little air drawn into the lungs results in oxygen-poor blood for your cells.*

Proper breathing uses the obliques and muscles of the abdomen and lower back to lower the diaphragm farther and allow for a much larger volume of respiration. The increased volume of air results in absorption in the *lower lungs,* maximizing the amount of oxygen that gets into the bloodstream.

Deep breathing not only increases oxygen to every cell of every tissue; it massages the internal organs, strengthens the lungs, activates the parasympathetic nervous system to leave us feeling more relaxed, reduces heart rate, lowers blood pressure, and deepens the connection between the mind and body. Deep breathing not only relaxes us; it gives us more energy and keeps the body thriving. Pain of all types can cause unconscious and dysfunctional muscle contractions, but slow, deep breathing encourages the muscles to relax, reducing discomfort.

> Many recent studies, including the largest one ever conducted on cannabis and lung health, have found that cannabis use increases lung volume. Toking actually strengthens the lungs.

Pranayama is a yoga term that means "regulation of breath." Pranayamas are yogic breathing practices that change one's physical, psychological, and energy state, usually slowing down the respiration and calming the nervous system.

For the following pranayama practices, keep the mind on the breath instead of other thoughts. When the mind wanders, come back to the sensory experience of breathing. It may not seem possible now, but once you cultivate more mindfulness, concentration, and relaxation, each breath will eventually become fascinating, a simple miracle (literally) right under your nose.

Deep Breathing Practice

By smoking or vaping cannabis, you're already doing a pranayama, which is diaphragm breathing. Let's deepen this practice:

1. Sitting comfortably, place a hand on your belly, keeping the shoulders relaxed.
2. Inhale as slowly and as deeply into your torso as you can without strain, feeling your belly press into your hand and your side ribs expand.
3. Exhale slowly. As you do, the hand moves toward the spine and the ribs move inward.
4. Enjoy a few more rounds, going slow and deep, using your hand as feedback.

This basic pranayama, called proper breathing, deep breathing, diaphragm breathing, belly breathing, or yogic breathing, is how we breathe during yoga poses, and how we should remember to breathe throughout the day. It may feel a little strange or unnatural at first, because the deep breathing muscles are usually weak from underuse. Making a habit of doing it more often strengthens the muscles and creates new neural grooves, so we can relearn the natural, functional, healthy breathing habits we were born with.

5. Now, take a deep breath again, being mindful to fill the belly and not puff up the chest.

6. Exhale, and as you do, open your mouth and let out an audible sigh, releasing the cares and worries of the day.

7. Continue to inhale deeply, and with each exhalation put yourself in a mood to relax.

8. You might internally repeat the phrases, "Mindful, I breathe in," as you inhale through your nose, and "Relaxed, I breathe out," on each exhalation, which can be open-mouth or through the nose. (Open-mouth exhalations tend to release tension even better. Try letting out a "hah" or "ah" sound as you let go!)

Placing awareness on the breath is the best way to become more present, and deep breathing is the best way to calm down the mind and become more relaxed.

Sometimes when we're doing breath work, unexpected emotional energy bubbles to the surface. Sometimes we suddenly tear up for no reason, or we find ourselves connecting with a painful memory that was buried long ago. It's natural to make sounds of release as we let go of built-up emotional tension. You don't necessarily have to know what the emotion is. Let whatever comes up come up, and release whatever wants to be released. We don't need to know what's in the trash bag; we just have to get it to the curb!

Yogic Three-Part Breathing Practice

When we smoke cannabis, we use the breath as the vehicle for the plant to enter our bodies. You can also use these breathing practices to deepen the cannabis high.

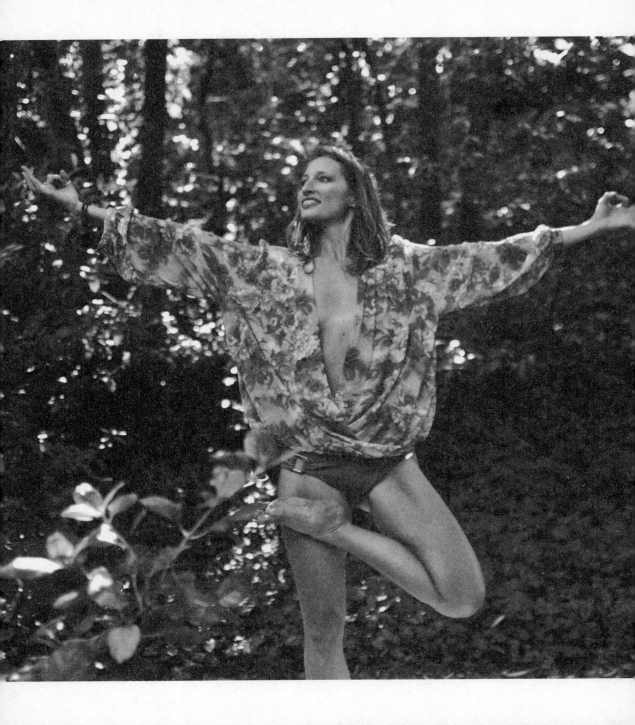

There's no shame in coughing! In fact, when you cough from smoking, you excite the muscles in your lungs, which causes the smaller air capillaries to open up. When this happens, more of the smoke or vapor enters your body. As my mom used to say, "You gotta cough to really get off."

One of the best pranayama practices is the Three-Part Breath. It starts with basic belly breathing, the deep breathing practice we already cultivate in yoga.

1. Feel the belly filling up as though you're inflating a balloon on your inhalation, and softly contract the abs to exhale.

2. On your next inhalation, add the second part. Fill your belly and then draw the same inhalation farther up into your rib cage, taking a somewhat longer in-breath and feeling it inflate more of the torso. Exhale, first from your chest and rib-cage area, then from your belly. Continue these two parts for a few more rounds.

3. To add the third part, which may be too strenuous for some, inhale and fill your belly, then expand your rib cage, and then take a sip of extra air up into the collar bones. Exhale from the top down.

If you have difficulty with all three parts, just do two or even one.

Next, take a few deep drags of cannabis vapor with one-, two-, or three-part breathing to bring the medicine deep into your tissues.

Congrats! You are an inspired inhaler at this point. And now you're finally ready to do what most people think of when they hear the word "yoga"—the poses!

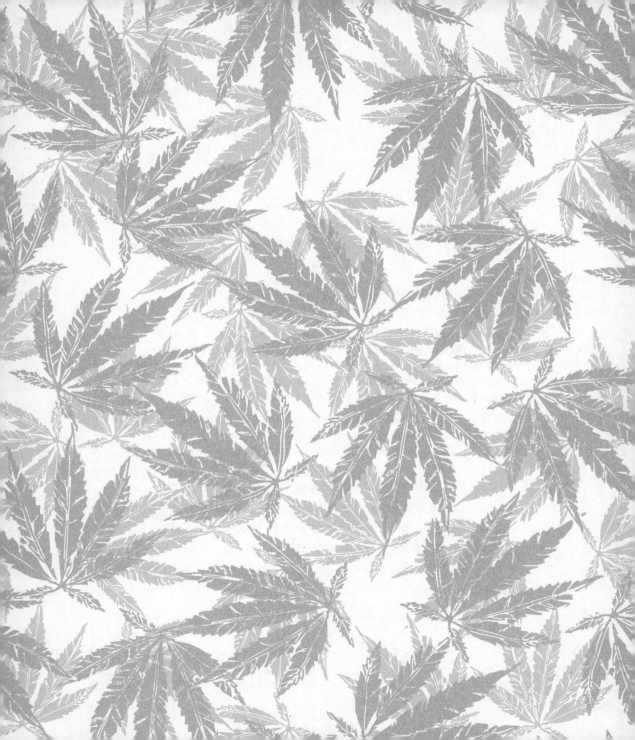

13

POSES FOR POTHEADS, PART 1:
Theory

ANCIENT YOGIS AND SAGES developed what we call "poses" as a way to tap into the energies of the sun and moon, various animals, and the natural elements of earth, water, fire, air, and ether, but poses were a very small part of yoga practice in early and medieval yoga. Traditionally the practice also included philosophy, cosmology, psychology, nutrition, ethical codes, and sexual practices, all rooted in mindful awareness and deeper spiritual states. According to yoga, harmonizing all of our many internal energies and emotions brings deep meditation, which brings enlightenment.

A lot can change over several thousand years. Today, yoga postures are known all over the world and, for the most part, they're regarded as the be-all and end-all of yoga, the dominant expression of practice. Breathing and mental practice are far less emphasized, and the other aspects (philosophy, ethics, sexuality, etc.) completely ignored.

As mentioned earlier, most of the poses we do today—actually a hybrid of Indian wrestling exercises and European gymnastics—were developed between one and two hundred years ago not as vehicles for the evolution of consciousness and the liberation of the soul, but as a form of *exercise* for health and well-being. I know it can be destabilizing to realize that the positions we've been practicing have little rootedness in ancient or even medieval practice, but I also find this information liberating. Humanity's vast collection of "yoga" poses offers numerous health benefits, and now we each can feel free to explore many different poses and styles, create modifications that suit our bodies, and question what we've been taught. We can also skip any pose we want from the "tradition," knowing it might not be any more "yoga" than, say, mindful hula-hooping.

I mention this to hammer home the point that yoga isn't necessarily what we think it is or has always been. It's important to dispel the preconceived notions you may have about yoga—for your enjoyment as well as your safety. I myself made some pretty harmful assumptions about what yoga should look and feel like. Luckily, you can learn from my mistakes!

Too Much of a Good Thing

We all like things that come easy to us. It's no wonder flexible dancer types with long limbs and mobile joints might be drawn to yoga. It's easy for them, and they look good doing it!

Me? I was pretty clumsy as a kid, extremely nearsighted, taller than most of my boy classmates, and always picked second-to-last in gym classes. (At least I was better than Steve.) After I got hit in the face with a volleyball and broke my glasses—twice—I gave up on athletics altogether, playing outfield (*way* outfield) in softball, daydreaming and writing my name in the dirt instead of playing the game. Most of my childhood was spent curled up reading.

Because I was clumsy and not into physical activities of any kind, my mom wasn't prepared for my reaction to the VHS yoga tape she gave me for Christmas in 1995—I loved it! We might not have been rich, but my mom always tried to get us a bunch of little gifts for under the tree. One of her strategies was to buy things from the bargain bin, so the tape was just another random stocking stuffer that I could take or leave, but I sure took it!

I especially liked the alone-time element of the practice, where nobody could judge me as I wobbled on one foot and moved into fun, strange shapes. Plus, the relaxation element came at just the right time for the emotional, anxious teenager I was fast becoming.

Best of all, I soon found that my gangly arms and long skinny legs made it easy to do postures that my friends found difficult. For the first time in my life, I managed to look long and graceful, contorting my spine to make grand swooping back bends and swan dives. I could even wrap my leg around my neck!

What I loved most was the Standing Forward Fold, where I could bend forward and not only touch my toes but tuck my palms *under my feet,* fingertips all the way to wrist creases. I did it all the time, thinking, "If flexibility is a good thing, then unbridled flexibility must be a great thing!"

After that first VHS tape, I continued doing any yoga I could find, which meant scouring yard sales in my rural town for books and videos. When I moved to Toronto for college, I would pop into studio classes here and there. Unless you stick with one studio (and I didn't), you don't really get direct, consistent attention from a yoga teacher. As a result, I had no one to tell me I was overdoing my favorite poses, making the same dysfunctional shapes with my body every single time I slid my palms under my feet. Rounding my spine was problem number one, and problem number two was that I was spending long periods with my spine in that shape, the *same shape* I spent lots of my childhood curled up reading in.

The interesting thing is, I didn't think I was pushing myself in my yoga practice. There was no pain. It felt relaxing. But it was *imbalanced.* I almost completely stopped doing any strengthening poses. "Why bother when it feels so good to stretch?" I thought.

Hypermobility means excessive range of motion, and it's not a good thing. A more accurate term, suggested by biomechanics teacher Katy Bowman, would be "joint laxity" or "hyperlaxity," because the connective tissues (ligaments and tendons) around a joint are *inelastic,* and as such do not return to their proper length after being overstretched.

People who are "hypermobile" often have muscles that are shorter and tighter than those with a regular range of motion. They *look* more flexible than they are because they distort their too-lax joints to achieve the shape—like me with my "graceful" Standing Forward Fold. Fifteen years of grand swan diving and forward hanging later, I woke up with back pain so bad I couldn't lean forward *at all*.

No Child Pose. No Standing Forward Fold. No drinking water out of the tap or putting on shoes normally or lying on my side to cuddle. And there was no apparent cause, other than the fact that I sat in a pretty slumped (but "normal") position in front of my computer the day before, then walked in flat, hard boots. I thought, "I'm healthy. I'm limber. I do yoga every day. This is nothing."

When I still had pain a few days later, I knew something was seriously wrong. Through something scientists call "mechanical creep," my many years of imbalanced yoga practice (and some bad postural habits off the mat) deformed the malleable connective tissues in my thoracic spine.

Unlike muscles, ligaments and tendons are *plastic*, not elastic. Once they're overstretched, they stay lax, and then they're not strong enough to hold the joints properly in place. The wrong muscles get recruited and overused as a result, bringing inflammation, tension, and pain to the area. Oh, and connective tissues can take up to two years to fully heal.

Worst of all, because I was hypermobile in that part of my spine, the connective tissues around my vertebrae were what had been moving all this time; so my back and hamstring muscles were *as inflexible as before*, despite countless hours dangling in the pose.

In yoga studios all across the country, people are trying to force themselves into certain shapes and as a result may be *damaging tissues*, even if, like me, they don't feel any pain at the time.

My story has two lessons:

1. Less is more. *Don't overdo any one thing.* Find the "minimum effective dose."
2. Strength and flexibility are *both* required for the health and functioning of the body.

Sometimes we do too much too soon when diving into something new, whether it's a weight-loss plan, a new relationship, or our exciting new yoga practice. It's a healthy awakening to realize we've been ignoring the body and now want to make amends with reparative action, but brutalizing it won't reverse the physiological effects of being sedentary and will probably cause injury. This is hard to resist. Notions about punishment and discipline are a part of our culture and may cause an unconscious tendency to push, obsessive control or discipline, or even masochism (allowing pain) to creep into our yoga practice.

MORE FLEXIBLE ≠ MORE SPIRITUAL

That gorgeous form you see doing conventional representations of yoga might be due to genetics that support that type of flexibility, a decade of gymnastics or ballet, or pushing it in yoga practice. A beautiful bending body or your ability to achieve a pose says zero about your character, your commitment, your potential, or even how well you are actually doing yoga. Remember, yoga is the yoking of the breath to the mind, not the stretching of the limbs for Instagram.

Even yoga itself has this heritage. Some Indian forms of yoga treat the body as illusory, a distraction or obstacle to self-realization. Some yogis performed severe body modifications to enhance their yoga practice, like swallowing several feet of cotton or cutting the flap of skin under the tongue. Some devout practitioners perform extreme austerities like holding their arm aloft for decades.

These intense yoga practices certainly impacted the teachers who came to the West. We might not be cutting our tongues, but are we dominating our bodies by ignoring the requirements of our connective tissues?

Ganja Yoga posture practice is mindful, full-body conditioning that focuses on ease, restorative flexibility, and relaxation. Knowing we are culturally conditioned to push and conquer, to see pain as "spiritual," or to become addicted to sensation, we need to be mindful of an inner urge to push beyond a joint's range of motion just to *feel something*.

It's natural to want to feel your body after you haven't been in touch with it. But if your yoga practice is to truly serve you and restore the body to its natural functioning, *intense sensation is not the solution.* Even if you don't injure yourself in the moment, constantly pushing or ignoring alignment needs will almost certainly lead to more dysfunction and greater bodily disconnection. Not to mention, overexertion causes the accumulation of lactic acid and other waste products in the tissues.

A "yoga body" is any body. A body that gets into certain shapes easily is not evidence of a yoga practice (the model in the yoga magazine may be a dancer or gymnast). And even if the strong, flexible body is the result of yoga poses, we have no idea what's going on inside. The tightness of your ass or your ability to touch your toes has zip to do with who you are as a person. Yoga is what happens on the inside.

Have a body? It's a yoga body!

Life is not about transcending the body. Life *includes* the body and all of its embodied experiences, sensations, needs, desires, and feelings. Although some yoga traditions disregarded the "meat body" as secondary to the spirit, others, such as Hatha Yoga and Tantra Yoga, consider care of the body to be one of the *pivotal practices.*

- Avoid chasing maximum intensity.
- Going beyond normal joint range is not virtuous.
- Play with becoming more sensitive to the subtle.
- Yoga is about exploring your edges, not pushing them.

It may be hard to resist "leaning into" strong sensations. If you already have a yoga practice and you suspect you're a sensation junkie (because you are numb and cut off from the connection with your body like the rest of our culture), this approach to yoga may take some *major unlearning*. If you're a Type A person, an achiever, a perfectionist, or a former dancer or gymnast, and especially if you identify as "flexible," this may be even more so.

Repeat this mantra anytime you want to extend just a bit farther: *Less is more, less is more, less is more, less is more.*

Cannabis helps this here. Awaken your inner relaxed stoner. Call in the archetypes of the Big Lebowski, Tommy Chong, a surfer dude chillin' in a hammock, a reclining Buddha, whatever helps you to *do less,* so you can find fascination with the subtle.

Yogic Strength

As I learned the hard way, strength is just as important as flexibility. But this is not the "strength" we're used to seeing. It's a quiet power, cultivated through holding bodily shapes our muscles aren't used to, not by lifting heavy weights. It's about having good alignment so our joints are getting appropriate and required loads, which gives them the mechanical stimulation to grow strong. As we take care to set the joints up properly each time we do restorative stretches or yoga postures, we ensure they remain healthy and strong.

To be healthy, muscles require *flexibility, strength,* and *relaxation.* Connective tissues around the joints require *mobility* (different joint movements) and gentle *strength training* with light loads (like bearing your own weight). They also require *release,* either via *yin*-style stretching or deep massage, to break up adhesions. Bones need to do the work they were meant to do; for example, leg bones require walking and squatting for strength. A complete movement practice also includes balance cultivation, which is a form of strength that will make aging go far more smoothly.

Having good form, varying the types of movements you do in yoga, doing yoga often, and supplementing your practice with regular walking is, in my opinion, all you need to be strong.

Now let's look at the not-so-secret ingredient that helps with all three components of healthy yoga practice: stretching. It's the simplest solution there is for flexibility, strength, and relaxation.

Stretchy Science Made Easy

When you put a cast on a broken body part to limit its movement, the immobilization brings a decrease in both muscle mass and bone mass. We don't need to wear a cast to experience this, however. Sitting the same way, walking the same way, sleeping the same way, not experiencing enough different joint positions throughout the day, and not moving enough in general all change the composition of the tissues the same way a cast on a broken arm does, as biomechanics guru Katy Bowman teaches.

When you chronically use your muscles in a limited and repetitive way, your body will respond to your habits and physically rearrange the muscle units (sarcomeres), so that you can more easily take that shape, even when you aren't intending to (ever have "Tyrannosaurus Rex arms" after being on the computer for many hours?).

Restorative Stretching

To stretch is to apply a load to the tissues that results in elongation. This keeps the muscles at their naturally long resting length and increases *flexibility,* which is the word for the healthy range of motion you have in your joints.

Restorative stretching brings a *necessary* weight and movement to the joints in ways that our modern lifestyle does not. For example, if we often type with our wrists bent at an angle, a restorative stretch moves the wrist in new ways. Restorative calf stretching corrects for the slight heel that most shoes (even men's) have. Restorative neck stretching is great after having the head forward to look at your phone all day.

Restorative movements look a lot less visually interesting or challenging than "yoga poses." However, a complete movement practice changes the position of all of the joints in the body in as many ways as possible and emphasizes the movements needed most. These movements restore the body's joints to their natural shape and functioning, returning the system to the way it would function if we didn't have our modern lifestyle of repetitive sitting, texting, typing; flat, hard pavement and thick-soled shoes; looking at screens at close range; and so on.

There's nothing wrong with yoga poses that don't offer restorative benefits. They're fun, and it's good to have fun. But if you're short on time, choose restorative stretches, poses, and practices that counteract the way you hold your body most of the time. Once more, mindfulness is key. Only *you* know what body parts need restorative movement!

HOW TO STRETCH

Sometimes it seems as though everything we know to be true has contradictory evidence. Whether the topic is saturated fat, cholesterol, caffeine, wine, jogging, or any number of other things, one study shows health benefits and another shows health harm. On top of this, radical new discoveries are being made every day (for example, about the properties of fascia, a web of connective tissue that covers every structure in the body). As with cannabis, there is just so much we don't know.

The same is true for stretching. There are no accepted standards for stretching, no one method or technique that has been shown to be superior, and lots of controversy and conflicting evidence. However, in the authoritative text *Muscle Pain*, researchers Siegfried Mense, David Simons, and I. Jon Russell state that stretching "by almost any means is beneficial."

Just like your relationship to cannabis, your relationship to stretching will be individualized, based on what works best for you.

Types of Stretches

Here's a rundown of the four types of stretches we do in my Ganja Yoga classes. Each of them works differently for relaxation, flexibility, joint mobility (flexibility plus strength), and overall good health.

DYNAMIC STRETCHING

Dynamic stretches are done with controlled, deliberate movements that slowly increase the range of motion of a joint. This is the best type of stretch for people new to movement, because it's the least likely to cause injury. It's also good for people who get bored easily, because there are a lot of different movements (though at the same time the repetitive movements help the mind relax).

Practices include stretches like rolling the shoulders down and back several times with the breath, wrist and ankle circles, easy flow-based yoga movements (Vinyasa), and slow warm-up drills done before exercising.

It's best to do dynamic stretches first thing in the morning to wake up the body and before other types of stretching or exercises.

HOW: Pick a body part that needs to be stretched and do eight to twelve slow, controlled repetitions of a joint rotation or movement, moving with the breath if that feels good. You can slowly pick up speed or increase the size of your movements as you warm up, though always move slowly with the neck. Do as many sets as it takes to reach your maximum range

Overstretching causes microscopic tearing of muscle fibers or connective tissues, increasing the time it takes for you to gain greater flexibility. Don't do it!

of motion in any given direction, but don't work your muscles to the point of fatigue. Rest afterward and feel the effects.

TIP: Mindful dynamic stretching can be its own yoga practice or a warm-up for other types of stretches or movements.

PASSIVE STRETCHING

Passive stretching uses your body weight (the support of your limbs or some other apparatus) to hold the stretch, so the muscles being stretched remain relaxed. This is what we usually think of when we hear the word "stretch," and it's also the main type of stretching done in yoga. Some examples of passive stretching include holding your arm, facing down, across your body with the opposite hand to stretch the biceps; pulling one finger down to stretch the hand; pressing the bottoms of your forearms against the sides of a doorframe to stretch the chest; hanging your foot off the side of a step to stretch your calf; or putting the arch of your foot in a yoga strap and pressing your leg out against the strap as you lie on your back to stretch your hamstrings. Passive stretching is good for people who want to stay still for a while and really relax in stillness.

I know you know this by now, but once more, just in case: intense stretching does *not* bring long, loose muscles. Once a muscle has reached its maximum length, attempting to stretch it beyond that point overextends the connective tissues, which are not elastic like muscle. Ligaments tear when stretched just 6 percent more than their normal length. Even if there is no tearing, loose overstretched connective tissues reduce stability in your joints, increasing your risk of injury later on.

When doing passive stretching, stay mindful and avoid intense sensation.

HOW: Do some dynamic stretching first to warm up. When doing a passive stretch, bring a lot of awareness (mindfulness) to your stretch. Find where the muscle first starts to feel new sensation and rest there for a while, breathing and feeling, and only increase the load when there is no resistance or tension. Breathe deeply, holding this type of stretch for twenty to sixty seconds or whatever feels good for you. Do one to three rounds of each stretch, with more frequent but shorter rounds if you're new to stretching.

More frequent stretching for shorter duration is the safest way to stretch. If you're new to stretching, worried about an injury, or out of shape, do two to five repetitions of each stretch, holding and breathing for ten to thirty seconds, with a rest in between each round. Your last round can be longer if that feels good.

Do passive stretches frequently so your body can adapt. Irregular stretching may cause injuries, even if it doesn't feel intense.

TIP: If you're using a prop (the floor, wall, yoga block, or other body part) to hold the stretch, see if you can completely relax the muscle that is stretching/elongating. If you're not using a prop, gently contract the opposite muscle. Remember, stretching might feel new or weird, but *there should never be pain or intense discomfort.*

YIN-STYLE STRETCHING

Because they are deformed more easily, the way we stretch (apply load for biomechanical benefit) tendons, ligaments, and fascia is different from the way we stretch our muscles. *Yin*-style is a type of passive stretching in which the loads are far less intense and held much longer, because they're designed for the connective tissues instead of the muscles. Because it is so low-intensity, the sensation is more like releasing than stretching. *Yin*-style stretching is good for people who want to stay in the Happy Baby Pose for a long, long time.

HOW: Be sure to do dynamic stretching beforehand to warm up. Practice *yin* stretches, such as the fan favorites Child Pose or Reclining Butterfly Pose, for two to three minutes, supported by props as needed, to give enough time for both the muscles and the tougher connective tissues to release. Breathe fully throughout, letting the exhalation take you deeper into surrender. Stay as long as you'd like!

TIP: The long holds allow the nervous system to really sink into the relaxation response. Come out of these postures very slowly, using other muscles to help you transition, so the ones you just opened can remain relaxed. Rest afterward and savor the sensation.

ACTIVE STRETCHING

The best way to truly change flexibility is to engage the brain and nervous system in the process of stretching. This ensures that the new sensory information from the muscles actually reaches the brain, which begins to "view" the muscles as long while training the nervous system to allow the stretch.

Active stretching, known by many names and with various similar techniques, involves contracting your muscles *as you elongate them* (or using resistance against the muscles as you stretch). This refreshes your brain's sensation of the muscle. You then spend a period of rest with the newly lengthened muscle fully relaxed, so the brain and nervous system register and allow this new, longer dimension. Although all types of stretches have unique benefit and are useful for everyone, active stretching is the most scientifically documented, so if you're short on time, stick to this kind.

STRETCHING FEELS GOOD

People who stretch regularly (and mindfully and with good alignment), find it feels good to stretch. The scientific reason why stretching reduces sensations of stiffness and soreness is not fully understood, but it is clear that once people develop the habit of stretching, they tap into the urge to stretch more and more often, the way cats stretch several times a day.

HOW: As with passive and *yin*-style stretching, it is best to do dynamic movements beforehand to warm up. Assume the position as you would for a passive stretch (like lying on your back with a strap around your foot and the heel pressing toward the sky to stretch the hamstrings). As you *tense* the stretched muscle (in this case, the hamstrings), for ten to fifteen seconds, resist against something else: the floor, wall, or another body part (in this case, the pull of your arms on the strap), breathing deeply. Engage the stretching/contracting muscles just enough that you can feel them as both *active* and *soft,* and make sure you're breathing. Next, relax the muscle for at least twenty seconds (lying with the leg down on the floor).

TIP: You can combine tools and do a passive stretch for another thirty seconds after an active stretch, followed by another twenty-second rest, for even greater flexibility gain.

Active stretching develops strength as well as flexibility, and builds a stronger connection between the sensory motor cortex of the brain and the muscles, bringing increased muscle control and coordination. It is said to be the most effective way to change flexibility.

Stretching and Pain

Torn muscle or connective tissue fibers heal at a shorter length than their relaxed resting length. This decreases flexibility in the injured area. Very light stretching of the injured muscles can realign disorganized connective tissue fibers, helping to rehabilitate scarred tissue. It should be far more gentle in sensation than you would normally feel in stretching (which is already very low intensity!).

Hold stretches around pain for about ten seconds, breathing slowly and deeply. Intense stretching of any kind may only make matters worse.

Sometimes even very gentle stretching is not appropriate when there are injuries to the tissues. If your pain and inflammation seem to get worse after even very gentle stretching, the tissue may not be benefitting from elongation. Stick to regular, slow, and gentle joint movements in the area (dynamic stretching), along with soft massage with topical cannabis and either a heating pad or cold compresses, whichever provides more relief.

Keep a soft awareness on your pain—not a harsh laser beam of attention, but a relaxed cloud of awareness. Allow your pain. Let it be. Facing what's real, fully experiencing the reality of what is, in every moment, is the key to yoga and most spiritual traditions. Continue to breathe deeply, perhaps sending the breath into the pain, releasing any mental tension and physical discomforts you are able to.

Suffering is often the catalyst for deep spiritual practice. Whether your pain is physical or emotional, let this be an opportunity to offer yourself deep care and comfort, a respite from the crazy world.

Emotional Pain, Physical Manifestation

My back pain was diagnosed as a simple "strain and sprain" (damage to both muscle and ligament). I was told it would heal in a few weeks. When months went by and it didn't, I started to become depressed. My new husband had to take care of me even though I had only just received my green card to start working. We didn't have the financial resources to keep me from feeling guilty for every "wasted" minute lying on the floor. I started to have thoughts like, "I can't have pain right now. I need to be seeing clients and running classes," and "I'm such a waste, just lying here when I need to be working."

He assured me I shouldn't stress, I should just rest and heal, but my mind couldn't drop it. "I shouldn't be having pain," I kept telling myself. "It's not a good time for this."

On top of the guilt I had for relying on someone who had already been so generous with me, I was feeling deep shame: "I am a yoga practitioner with two decades of practice. If anybody, shouldn't *I* be free of pain?"

And then, layers upon layers: "Dee! You are a yoga teacher. You shouldn't be judging yourself for feeling pain! Why can't you be more compassionate with yourself? It's not very spiritual of you to not accept reality!!"

And so the cycle of internal abuse continued, and naturally this emotional suffering caused more intensity in my chronic pain, which caused more despair, and then more self-judgment.

Even though I knew all of this intellectually, I still got sucked into it. I had the mindfulness part down pat, but that just meant being aware of how my inner voices were hurting me.

After some time, fortunately, there was only so deep I could spiral, and something turned the depression around. I let myself *be in pain*. I let myself be taken care of. I shed the guilt. And slowly—very, very slowly—my back healed, and I found myself spending less time on the floor and more time creating my website and meeting with clients.

Modern medical science finally recognizes the important role the mind-body connection plays in our health and well-being. Our thoughts and feelings create biomechanical changes in the brain that impact our emotional and physical well-being, including our perception of both pain and stress.

Further, scientists have recently found a nerve pathway between the adrenal glands (the organs that respond to stress) and the motor areas of the brain, specifically the part of the brain that maps out our torso. What their findings show is that doing postural work for the core, as in yoga and Pilates, positively impacts our stress response through neural connections.

It isn't easy to be mindful and compassionate, a being of light, when you're beaten down by chronic pain. I had nearly two decades of yoga practice under my belt when mine hit and I descended into as much darkness as anyone. (Perhaps even more. Remember, my negative thoughts were self-judgments because I "should have been doing better inner yoga"!)

When dealing with pain, mindfulness of all emotions, thoughts, associations, and inner judgments is crucial. See it all. Witness how you talk to yourself, all the little voices. This is true for everyone, and especially when managing pain.

Developing an even larger capacity for nonjudgmental self-awareness is the key to noticing pain-related negative thought patterns.

Allowing yourself to feel and express emotions keeps them from being lodged in your tissues as pain. When we're able to express and release our thoughts and feelings, the brain secretions return to homeostasis. If uncomfortable emotions aren't resolved or expressed, homeostasis is not attained, and emotional tension gets stored physically.

If you are managing chronic pain, yoga presents an opportunity to befriend the body. Any fear, anger, sadness, guilt, or other emotion that comes up as you allow and surrender into physical pain is *normal*.

Breathe and feel. You are loved.

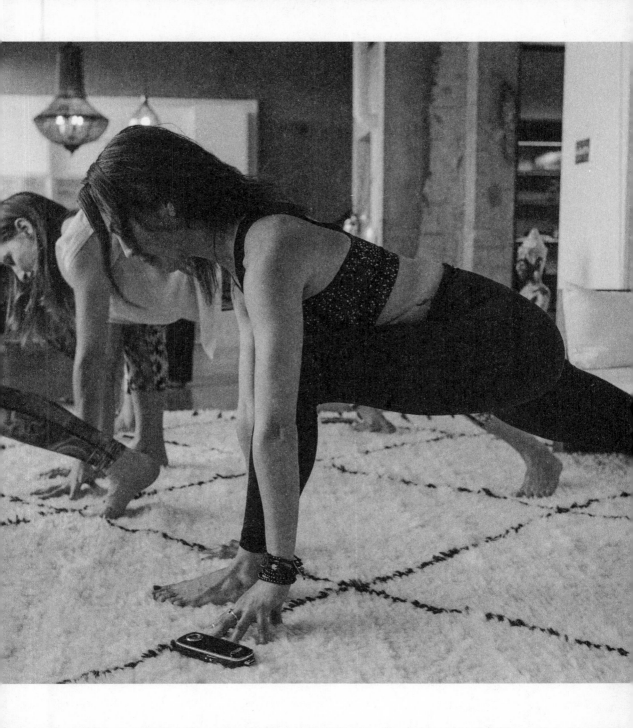

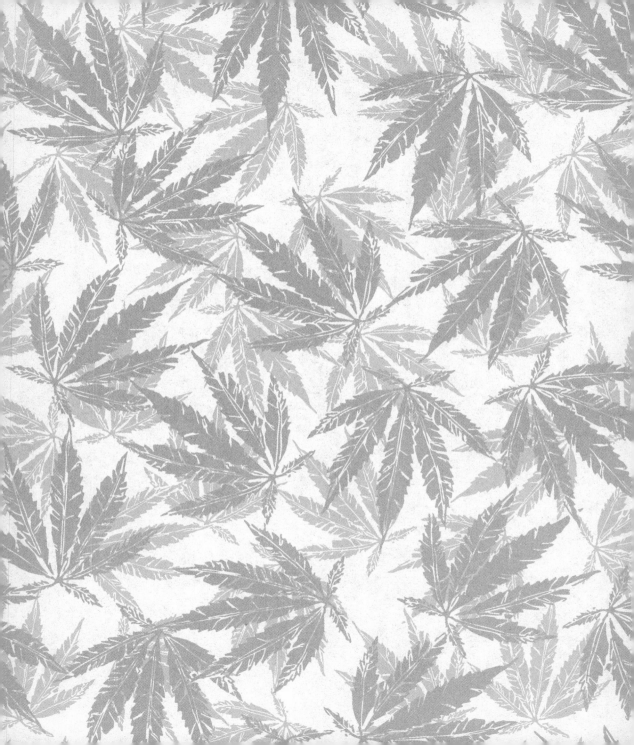

14

POSES FOR POTHEADS, PART 2:
Practice

HOPEFULLY MY STORY HAS INSPIRED you to not ignore strength, healthy alignment, and a balanced approach to your yoga practice. Bringing mindfulness to the human urge to push, compete, reach, rush, and accomplish will take you *so very far*. However, there may also be movement blind spots that harm your yoga practice, even when you're practicing nonstriving.

Movement Blind Spots

A *movement blind spot* is a dysfunctional habitual movement pattern. When we move in the same way a lot, the brain "zones out," and our movements become unconscious. If the movements are healthy, this is a useful adaptation. It's a waste of resources for the brain to "see" every movement required by the arm to brush our teeth, for example. However, if there are dysfunctions in how we repeatedly walk, stand, sit, text, or do yoga poses, the blind spot will not be useful because it will hide a bad habit.

As you know, if you habitually put your joints into the same position, this blind spot will eventually cause tissue dysfunction and pain. Although there are many ways yoga practitioners can be "blind" to their unique movement patterns, the *ribs* and the *pelvis* are the two most common blind spots I see in my classes.

MOVEMENT BLIND SPOT NUMBER ONE: THE RIBS

In the back, your ribs are attached to your backbone. In the front they are attached to your sternum, or breastbone. When you thrust your front ribs forward and up, your back arches. When you drop the ribs down onto the belly, the spine may feel rounded, but it's actually *neutral*.

In our culture, it is thought desirable to "stand tall," with the shoulders down and back (perhaps influenced by military practices). As a result, we have a bunch of people (myself included) popping the front ribs up and *deforming* the spine. We walk and sit and do yoga like that, feeling proud of our good posture.

Over time this unconsciously repeated deformation will inevitably become tension, pain, and tissue damage in the upper or middle back (or else will be compensated for elsewhere in the body). Yikes!

MOVEMENT BLIND SPOT
NUMBER TWO: THE PELVIS

Whether doing forward-folding movements, sitting, standing, or walking, the position of the pelvis is crucial to healthy spine alignment. Your pelvis (hip bones on either side, flat bony triangle of the lower spine, and pubic bone in the front) holds the lower back in place. If the top of your pelvis always tilts backward while you sit, so the tailbone goes under you and the pubic bone moves closer to the belly button, your lower back loses its natural curvature.

Similarly, if you don't tilt the pelvis forward (pubic bone away from belly button, tailbone back behind you), in forward-folding poses, the roundedness of your lower back can permanently deform the tissues of the spine or pelvic floor.

Your yoga teacher is there to offer favorite poses and ideas and to help you learn to listen to your own body. By all means, inform your teacher about your major health issues or injuries, but remember, you are the person responsible for your well-being. Take time to learn about your health issues, so you can make modifications for them to ensure a complete movement practice. Marry that information with mindfulness, intuition, and plenty of patience.

The reason we unconsciously tuck the pelvis under is chronic sitting. Short hamstrings and calves are the result of flexing the hips and knees to sit all the time, and the short muscles on the backs of the legs pull the pelvis back, out of alignment.

Another issue is letting the pelvis thrust forward with the weight in the front of the foot. If the hips remain straight on top of the heels, you'll know you're not displacing the pelvis forward *or* back.

All right, grab your doobie, yoga mat, and a full-length mirror if you have one—it's time to play!

Practice: The Ribs and Pelvis

Stand, in front of a mirror if possible, feet facing forward, hip-distance apart.

Thrust up and then lower your front ribs, seeing and feeling the effect it has on your spine. Try to keep your pelvis and hips neutral (both hip bones facing the front wall equally, and the floor equally). Keep the pelvis still.

When the ribs are thrust up, you can poke a little bit of your finger under the bottom ones; when they're flat, you can't. Can you see the ribs move in the mirror? Can you see how the upper/mid back contorts out of neutral as the ribs thrust up?

It might not be much movement, but the strain it causes the spine can be significant. Spend some time noticing the effect of this small postural habit, perhaps undressed so you can see your back and front ribs when you are standing with your side to the mirror.

Now, place your hand on your lower chest, where the ribs meet, and push your hand against your sternum to move it toward the belly. *That's* what we're going for.

> Notice how the common instruction "shoulders down and back" thrusts your ribs up. Although we want the shoulders to be away from the ears, keeping the shoulders down and the same distance apart is the best alignment position.

In every yoga pose, and throughout our days, we want to keep the ribs flat on the belly and in toward the spine.

Notice if you have this blind spot and thrust your ribs up because you were taught it was "good posture." Let the ribs be where they're supposed to be, and don't squeeze your shoulder blades together.

Now slowly lift your arms up in front, as high as you can *without lifting the ribs*. See where you are in the mirror? Never lift higher than that to attain a "yoga pose." This is your shape, for now. Resist hard-core back bends if it results in lifting the ribs. Bring light to this blind spot. As the shoulders get more flexible, you'll be able to lift the arms higher without distorting your spine.

Okay, bring the arms back down and try circling the arms to the sides and up—again, without lifting the ribs off the belly or arching the spine. Tight shoulders may prevent the arms from being vertical, and that's okay.

Now, shake out the arms and become aware of your hips and pelvis. Once more, standing, place your hands on your hips. Your feet should be far enough apart so that they are directly beneath the hips and facing forward. Your legs should be straight, and your ribs and shoulders are *where*?

Keeping the ribs down and still, begin to mindfully "tuck" and "untuck" your tailbone. When it's tucked, it is between your legs. Your legs are straight, and you have the tail of a sad or scared dog. Now, untuck your tailbone, without forcing or straining your back muscles. Do a few more rounds. As you tuck, you feel the pubic bone move toward the belly button; as you untuck, you feel the pubic bone move away.

Feel how your lower back gets unnaturally flattened when you tuck and resumes its natural curve again

> The only time we tuck the tailbone is when we're doing back-bending yoga poses like the Cobra, Sphinx, and Camel. In these we let the tailbone move like that of a sad dog and let the lower back flatten. Similarly, we tuck when we're reaching up to get something heavy from overhead.

when you untuck. (When you are untucked, you don't have to exaggerate the curve; just *allow* it.)

Whenever you can, in sitting, standing, lying down, and doing yoga, maintain a neutral (untucked) pelvis.

It's quite challenging to keep both the ribs and pelvis neutral; when you adjust one, the other wants to change. Play with it a bit longer while you are standing, keeping the weight in the heels, the head back so the ears are directly over the shoulders, the legs straight, and the belly soft. *Make sure you're breathing.*

As weird as this may all feel at first, this is good alignment from the perspective of biology and physics. We all have bad habits that pull us out of it, but over time restorative yoga practices and cannabis-enhanced awareness can bring us back.

Do a few more rounds, then shake your whole body. *Shake, shake, shake, shake, shake!*

Now stand normally for a moment and rest.

Now play with these two blind spots while sitting, kneeling on all fours, and lying on your back with your knees bent, feet on the floor. Pay attention to your ribs and pelvis in each position and in all your yoga poses going forward.

> Awareness is the first step to making any change.

Strike a Pose

Every tissue in our body needs movement to remain healthy. We were created through evolution to be in motion. Our early ancestors walked vast distances to find food. Movement is an essential part of healthy functioning for all animals.

When you move your body in new ways, your brain gets novel sensory input and creates new neural pathways to perform the movements. This is called *neuroplasticity,* the brain's ability to adapt. Learning new things, moving in different ways, walking barefoot on various textures, experiencing new cultures, making love in many positions, and other such experiences keep the brain adaptive.

It is for this reason I am reluctant to spew out the "how to" for the few dozen common yoga poses that you see in most studios across the world. There are countless videos, classes, and articles online with the same information I'd give you. What I want to teach is that *all kinds of mindful movement* can be useful and relaxing while high—as long as it feels good for your body (and you follow basics of good alignment).

Your yoga practice can be whatever you want it to be.

How you do your yoga is a lot more important than *what* yoga you do.

Having said that, the following are some of my favorite poses and restorative stretches. Consider them springboards to propel you toward discovering the yoga-inspired movements *your body* most wants. No matter what you do, mindfulness and deep breathing are the most important aspects.

But first, how are your cannabis levels?

Perhaps you'd like some CBD tincture to offset pain or anxiety. Or maybe you'll take a heavy indica edible, so after a few poses you can drift off to sleep. If you're chillin' out, stretching with friends, perhaps passing a beautiful pipe is where it's at.

Do whatever you need to do to enhance your practice, or just say, "Not right now," if you'd like. The "what, how, and how much" part is individualized and vastly varied in effect. Be sure to warm up before doing deep stretches or challenging poses, especially if you do your yoga

Poses for Potheads

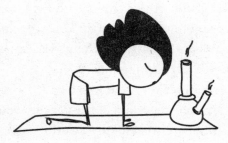

TABLE POSE

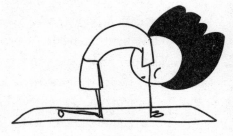

CAT POSE

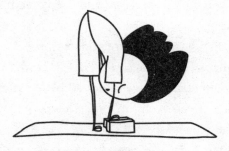

SUPPORTED STANDING
FORWARD FOLD

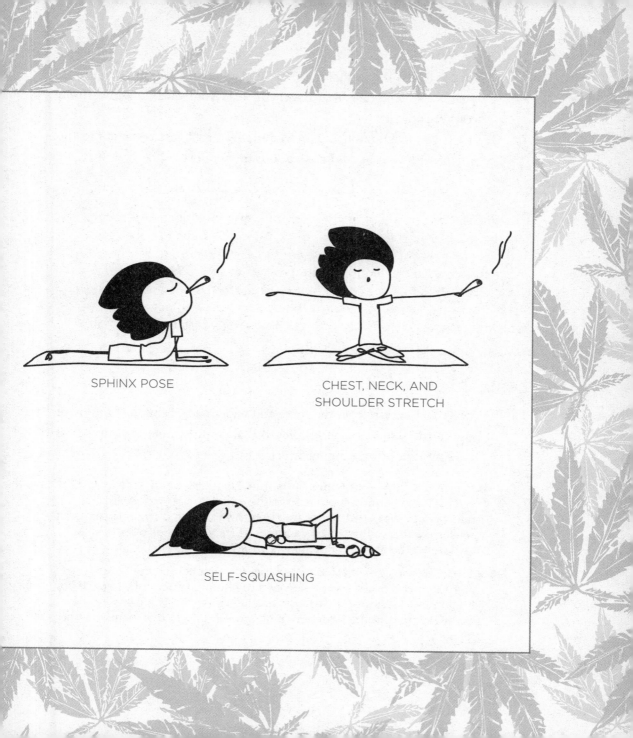

SPHINX POSE

CHEST, NECK, AND
SHOULDER STRETCH

SELF-SQUASHING

practice first thing in the morning. Joint rotations and other controlled dynamic stretches are best; match them to your breath as a warm-up breathing practice.

If you feel too much pain to do movements, just rest and breathe, perhaps with your hands on your body for comfort.

The *breath* is as important as the body in every yoga posture. Proper breathing is required to get all the gains from a stretch. It relaxes the muscles and nervous system, increases blood flow throughout the body, and helps to move out lactic acid and the other byproducts of exercise. Use the breath to help you enter and exit the stretch or pose. Take slow, relaxed breaths deep into the belly when stretching, exhaling whenever you want to take the sensation deeper or really release tension.

TABLE POSE

The Table Pose stretches the spine and upper back, bringing yummy release to the shoulders, neck, forearms, abdominal muscles, and hands. This simple pose is one of my favorites.

1. On all fours, have your hands under the shoulders, open wide or resting on fists. If the hands are open, have the middle finger parallel to the sides of your mat, the thumbs pointing toward each other, and the wrist creases parallel to the top of your mat. Have your knees directly under the hips, so the arms and thighs are straight and vertical.

2. Check the two common movement blind spots: untuck the tailbone, so the belly drops down and relaxes and the bum tilts naturally back. If you sit a lot, this may not feel very natural. Don't be shy! Then, ensure the ribs at the front of the body are gently moving up to the spine and onto the belly.

3. Press the hands or fists firmly into the floor so the shoulders are "locked" in their sockets, moving down and away from the ears, keeping them over the wrists.

4. Drop your head, relax the back of your neck, and soften your belly, pressing firmly into the hands to soften the shoulders. Breathe.

Awareness

- Feel tension in the shoulders and neck melt away as you press the hands into the floor. Let each exhalation soften the neck.

- Let the belly be soft, letting the organs in your torso relax down. Feel the sensation of release here for a few breaths.

- Spend a few breaths with the awareness at the hands, wrists and forearms, fronts of hips (hip flexors), and the backs of thighs/bum.

> You can also begin small, dynamic stretches in this pose, changing the weight distribution in the arms, and gently moving the head to introduce new loads to the tissues.

CAT POSE

The Cat Pose provides flexion to the spine without the intense load that a forward fold can bring. It's an awesome way to stretch and engage the upper back muscles, which often go neglected as we drive and type, especially if you do dynamic movements from within the pose.

1. When you're ready, get on all fours in the Table Pose, checking all the required alignment points. Close your eyes and, before moving into Cat, feel your whole body. Notice the weight distribution on the hands, shoulders, and knees on the left and right sides. Notice where you might have tension. When doing yoga, we always bring awareness to the body first, and then add conscious breathing and movement.

2. For the Cat Pose, press the palms or fists firmly into the floor and begin to arch your spine like a Halloween cat, keeping your shoulders forward, right over the hands. At the same time, curl your tailbone under (tucking it, which we don't usually do, but in this case, the load is very minimal).

3. Breathe and play with shifting your body weight, a little forward, a little back, a little left, a little right. We're looking for small, subtle sensations and inner connection. Keep your arms straight.

Awareness

- In your upper back is probably where you're going to be feeling this, so send your breath and awareness there.

- Notice any difference you might feel on the left and right sides.

- Allow an open-mouth exhalation, and see if you can let go of accumulated tension in the shoulder area.

> *Asanas,* poses, are a combination of attention (awareness), breath, and minimal effort. Obviously, some muscles get engaged in a posture, but there should eventually be such a feeling of ease, lightness, and surrender that it's as if no effort is being made.

CHEST, NECK, AND SHOULDER STRETCH

The Chest, Neck, and Shoulder Stretch can be done anytime, anywhere. I do it when I'm on work calls; I turn on speakerphone and let go of the strain that texting and typing bring to my shoulders, chest muscles, forearms, and hands. Tight shoulders and pectorals pull on the upper back, causing it to stoop. You might lift your ribs to hide it, but better is to spend some time doing this pose each day to reduce mechanical creep (the name given to deformed tissues, not my ex-boyfriend's punk band).

1. Sit or stand with the pelvis and ribs neutral and extend the arms out to the sides, as high as ninety degrees from the body, extending long from the elbows. Turn the palms up if that's comfortable, and breathe, letting the shoulders soften.

2. After some time, drop the head if that feels good, keeping the upper back from rounding. The shoulders are down and *broad,* the front ribs are on the belly, and the tailbone is untucked. Breathe.

3. When you're ready to release the pose, inhale and use the upper back muscles to slowly lift your head back up, ears gently moving back over the shoulders. Float the arms down to rest. Close your eyes and notice what you feel.

Awareness

• Hang out here and breathe, scanning the body, noticing whenever you're holding unnecessary tension and letting it go. Let the cannabis deepen your sensitivity, inner awareness, and capacity for embodied pleasure.

Flexibility is about the nervous system as much as the muscles. Stretching gives the nervous system repeated exposure to the sensation of the muscles elongating, so it will allow lengthening of your muscles.

As K. Pattabhi Jois said, "Body is not stiff; mind is stiff."

SUPPORTED STANDING FORWARD FOLD

Spreading the vertebrae and the disks between them away from each other brings suppleness to the back, increasing the range of movement in the spine and reducing pain.

1. Stand with the feet head-width apart facing a wall, the back of a chair, or two yoga blocks on the floor in front of you. The more flexible your hamstrings are, the lower your prop can be.

2. Have your weight in your heels, and place your hands on your hips. Keep the *neutral curve* of the lower back by ensuring the pelvis stays neutral (pubic bone down, tailbone up); then hinge forward from the hips without bending the knees or letting the pelvis or spine change *whatsoever*.

3. Place your hands on your prop, shoulder-width apart, shoulders moving down your back, tailbone gently rising as you move the hips back and lengthen the spine. Let the belly soften as you guide the ribs back to the spine and belly. Breathe.

4. To release, bring your hands back to your hips, your weight into your heels, and then slowly come back to standing with *the same neutral spine* and your core gently engaged.

DON'T ROLL UP THE SPINE!

In the end I'm grateful to my alignment sloppiness, because through it I learned healthy biomechanics and can now help others. I was often taught to "roll up through the spine" when coming back to standing from the Standing Forward Fold. Although moving the joints in all positions keeps them nourished, slowly rolling up from a folded position unnaturally places the weight of the upper back, rib cage, and head on the disks of the spine.

Instead, come up to standing by bringing the hands to the hips and inhale as you unhinge the spine from the hips, weight back in the heels, lifting the back as one unit, and maintaining its natural shape by staying neutral in the ribs and pelvis.

Awareness

- Let the upper back release as you feel your whole body.

- Be aware of the ribs and pelvis blind spots and anywhere else you might be asymmetrical or holding tension.

- Notice if you're holding the breath or straining.

SPHINX POSE

The Sphinx Pose is good after being on the computer all day. Plus you can puff as you recline in it, perhaps putting your joint into a French-style cigarette holder and tapping into your classy inner Cleopatra.

1. Come to a resting position on your tummy and come up on the elbows, placing them beneath the shoulders, or slightly more forward if comfortable. Your forearms are parallel to the sides of your mat, palms facing down.

2. Pull down through the elbows to gently lift the belly and chest off the floor. Press the pubic bone toward the floor to open the spine and engage your core, the deepest part of your lower belly and pelvis. Keep the rest of your body relaxed and breathe.

3. Bring in mindfulness, everything you know yoga to be. At the same time, have a sense of spiraling the elbows inward while pressing down with the palms and forearms to lengthen the front and back of the torso, keeping the shoulders down. Let the legs extend behind you, your feet about head-width apart, pressing down gently.

4. Close your eyes and feel your belly rising and falling as you continue to breathe. For a variation, let the head softly drop down, releasing the neck.

5. When you're ready to release, engage the muscles between the shoulder blades to slowly lift the head back up.

Awareness

- Whenever your mind wanders from the sensations of your body and the slow deep breathing, gently bring your awareness back to the practice and your experience. Remember, this mental aspect is as much a part of yoga as the physical aspects.

- With each exhalation, let yourself relax more and more, scanning your whole body for places that could soften as the breath leaves your body.

BONUS: SELF-SQUASHING

Every structure in the body is covered in a web of connective tissue called fascia. Fascia encapsulates and connects the organs, muscles, tendons, ligaments, joints, nerves, bones, and blood vessels, allowing them all to slide without friction.

When we don't move an area of the body enough, especially after an injury, the fascial tissues can bind together, causing sensations like knots, ropes, or gristle. This is especially the case when we're dehydrated.

Emotional tension that hasn't been expressed is thought by some theorists to be stored in the physical tissues of the fascia. It's been theorized that the body "swallows" these feelings as a kind of compensation mechanism, so the mind doesn't have to suffer.

Emotions are biologically real, and they make chemical changes to the body. When they get held instead of being expressed, they eventually cause physical tension, pain, and changes to body structures that limit mobility and functioning.

Ever feel extra tender or emotional after a deep massage or a yoga class with lots of long-held stretches? If so, you may have been releasing some past anger, fear, or sadness from the fascia.

BOREDOM

Mindfulness is what keeps yoga interesting. A pose you may have done hundreds of times brings something new to your awareness every time you do it, if you practice it fully, rest in it, and feel the nuances. As they say, you never step in the same river twice.

If boredom arises during your stoned yoga practice, cultivate beginner's mind. Find something interesting in your body and mind to become aware of. Cannabis makes this easier. Let the plant heighten what's showing up for you: the pulse, flow, buzz, heaviness, lightness, expansion, release, or whatever else it is. Let the weed make it fascinating.

Know this too: Boredom is also a part of the practice, a part of being alive, something to mature around. In this regard, I remember a teacher saying, "A yoga pose begins the moment you want to get out of it."

If you find holding easy poses, doing gentle stretches, breathing, being present, and just being all too boring compared to powerful, hard, fast-moving yoga, it probably means you need it to balance out your more active practice.

Nobody's saying stop doing your power yoga, weight lifting, or running, because ignoring yang is just as imbalanced as ignoring yin, as I learned.

However, be sure to do less sometimes. Your nervous system will thank you.

Although talk therapy has its benefits for releasing emotional tension, by the time unexpressed tensions are buried in the tissues, only physical release techniques can remove them. The good news is we don't need to know the content of the tension we're shedding. Letting go physically brings palpable release and expansion on the emotional level while dramatically increasing functionality in the tissues.

Every time you release these stuck tissues, they undergo biochemical and mechanical changes that create more efficient movement patterns, giving you the opportunity to repattern unconscious, chronic holding patterns (your blind spots). Although stretching (especially long-held, low-intensity *yin*-style stretches) can remove adhesions, self-massage techniques with foam rollers and other tools like squash or tennis balls are the best way to return suppleness and mobility to the fascia.

Self-squashing is my absolute favorite yoga move!

1. Using one or two tennis or squash balls or a foam roller, place the body part on the balls and let your body weight apply deep pressure to your muscles and fascia, resting on the very tender spots. Relax *into* the sensation as you soften the tissues over the roller or balls. Breathe deeply, and make sure you're not introducing tension into other body parts.

2. Press your "hot spots" firmly into the balls or roller, or move in small circles or side to side. Stay for three to five breaths. (Move at a speed of about one inch per second if you're on the roller.)

Awareness

- Feel the sense of melting your tissues instead of contracting them.

- Be aware of any emotional energy that comes up. Whatever comes in, let it in. Whatever comes out, let it out.

Sequencing

Every single time you practice yoga, it will look different. Sometimes you'll do a bunch of different yoga poses, and sometimes you'll do some dance-style movements and then a pose or two. Sometimes you'll focus on restorative stretching, and other times you'll practice harder, more bad-ass postures or even flows.

Sometimes you'll do the same sequence as yesterday, but it will feel totally different because of how much you slept, the mood you're in, the tunes you're playing, or the type, amount, and method of ganja used.

The structure and sequence of *your* practice is up to you. In *my* Ganja Yoga practice, every couple of poses are followed by a rest, so I can feel the effect of the movement on my body. I usually do thirty minutes of restorative movements in the morning, about an hour of passive stretching and *yin* poses (and foam rolling) in the evening, and many little stretches throughout the day.

No matter what we do, we always end with meditation, the fruit of our movement practice.

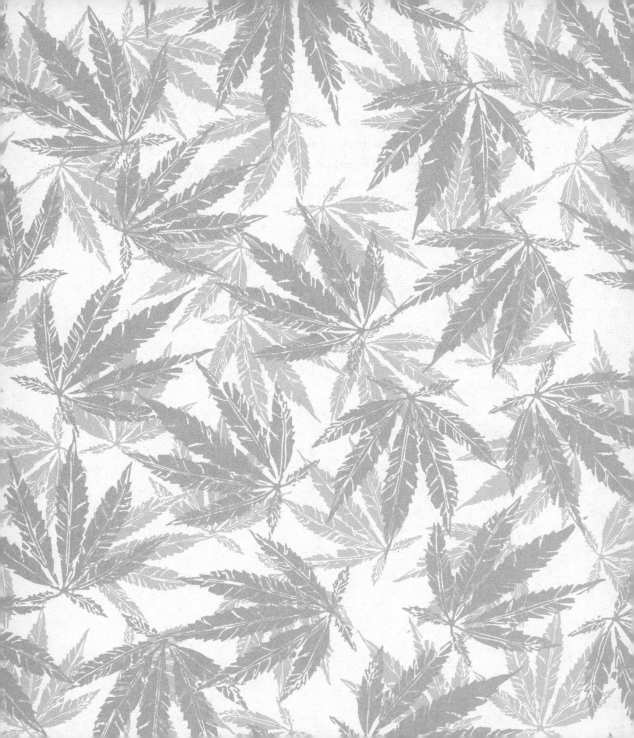

15

MARIJUANA MEDITATIONS

YOU KNOW THE PRACTICE OF YOGA has mindfulness as the foundation, followed by proper breathing, then restorative movements that bring strength, balance, flexibility, and relaxation. After movement comes stillness, which leads to meditation.

When most people think "yoga" nowadays, they envision handstands, beautiful back bends, vigorous Vinyasa flows, and hard-ass balance postures. We're mesmerized by the promise of being able to contort our bodies into impossible shapes, yet every yoga book, guru, and lineage would agree: we soar highest in our spiritual practice when we lie on our backs, eyes closed, going beyond the body, beyond the mind even.

The VHS tape my mom bought me may have been my introduction to yoga, but the meditation books I quickly started buying at yard sales were what got me interested in the spiritual promise of the Eastern practice.

After just a few *minutes* of meditation, people experience increased feelings of relaxation and improved cognitive function. And, because meditation *permanently rewires the physical matter of the brain*, it can enhance happiness levels *long-term*.

The Sanskrit definition of *yoga* is "the suspension of the movements of the mind." Meditation is the act of finding stillness on the outside so you can find silence on the inside.

The practice takes many forms. They all encourage us to look inward, so we can begin to fully see the workings of the mind. We see how the many "mental movements" keep us away from the present moment and strengthen the sense of an individual ego, which causes us suffering.

With time, the wildness of the mind begins to quiet down (we learn to suspend the movements), and a deep experience of inner peace can be found. **We come to realize that peace and love are the truth of our existence, not scarcity and competition.**

Once we experience this realization, disappointments, limitations, worries, and other suffering are markedly diminished, slowly but surely. This is the goal of yoga, and it's only possible when we are able to transcend the ordinary ways we experience our body and mind.

Our culture does not encourage us to do practices to quiet or dis-identify with the egocentric mind. In fact, we are bombarded by constant mental stimulation and agitation. We boast about how busy we are, how many things we have going on at once. The truth is that many of us are stressed out, overwhelmed, angry, judgmental, afraid, disconnected, or depressed. Instead of feeling as though we are a vital part of the cosmic whole, many of us feel like crap. Just tired little hamsters going nuts on the wheel, running in circles. Many of us are unable to stop and *rest*, let alone develop the patience and perseverance to train the mind to be *quiet* so we can tap into our so-called divine nature.

I get it. I've been there. *I am there.* All the time. I lose the thread, I fall off the horse. I get swept up in all the superficial chatter and ego-based fears of the mind. I get acquisitive. I care about getting "Dee" what she wants. I fear "Dee" will lose what's hers. Instead of seeing my place within the universe, abundant and secure, I often identify as a separate being.

It isn't easy to do otherwise. Our whole economy operates on the basis of our feeling separate, unique, individual, and selfish. It then becomes "normal" to strive to get ahead as an individual, to care only about what's ours (our own family, our own house, our own health, our own country), and to try to acquire as much (money, wealth, status, security, love) as we can before the clock inevitably runs out.

Yoga states that *all* negative inner states arise because we think we're separate from the rest of the cosmos, from each other, from the whole. If we are only our identity and body, we are left with the fact that when the body and identity die, we no longer exist. This is what makes death a terrifying thing. Meditation practices help us remove egoic attachment to the body and identity and ultimately help us shed this unconscious fear of death. We then become less obsessed with reliving things that happened and planning how we'll respond to things that may happen. We bring stillness to the fluctuations of the mind, so it can rest in a timeless state of pure being. When we are in this state, we can feel our limitless potential and our sense of importance to the whole.

By tapping into this feeling of unity-consciousness often enough, the cells of our brain start to create a groove, making it easier to attain this each time thereafter. **The mind is plastic: as you think, so you become.**

Easier said than done, though, right?

Why Meditation Feels So Hard

Meditation grants us the time to go beyond our external entanglements to a place of relaxation and deep inner connection. Even though this is our natural state, it takes practice to shed the layers of conditioned tension that keep us from experiencing it.

If you have tried meditation and it was hard because your mind was really busy, know that this is *normal*. It isn't ideal, it isn't *natural*, but it is normal. Avoiding meditation because the mind is busy is like not stretching the limbs because you're not flexible. You do stretches precisely because you're not flexible!

Moving through the "it's hard" feeling is part of meditation practice. See if you can be compassionate and patient with your busy mind, gently bringing it back every time it wanders off.

Meditation can also feel challenging because it is boring at times. Nothing seems to be happening. The trick to spirituality is to do practices to help awaken to our true nature without grasping or avoiding any one part of reality. If it's boring, be with the boredom. Cultivate willpower.

Over time, meditation helps us to experience peace, bliss, and contentment, no matter what is going on in our life.

Finally, meditation can feel hard because it puts us in touch with the underlying mental tensions that cause our dissatisfaction and irritability. We come to realize that most of our thinking is just a bunch of unconscious reactions, a bunch of negative, silly bullshit.

The meditation experience is about looking into the abyss within. It's not about feeling only happiness, but seeing *all* your thoughts, habits of mind, and assumptions, and how they cause you suffering. Most people understand that childhood disappointments remain in our psyche and influence our responses to the world, but if we can view them with compassion and detached awareness, they won't control us anymore. This is part of the healing benefit of meditation. By becoming aware of all that is, *including parts of ourselves that we find hard to accept,* those shadow aspects of egoic consciousness are effortlessly shed. Of course meditation feels hard to the ego—it doesn't want to be released!

When our mind becomes increasingly untroubled and increasingly loving, our world will be experienced in the same light. This is the heaven on earth that yoga is said to bring.

Instead of only dealing with the exterior situations that lead to conflict, stress, and agitation, a yoga practitioner looks within to find the causes of unhappiness. Altering only external situations simply treats the symptoms. With meditation, the personality and behaviors take a more positive direction, changing the internal feeling to the point where the external influence no longer holds the same power.

Joy, peace, power, and well-being are cultivated during meditation, and this further scrubs tensions from the mind. The two-part practice of seeing and releasing dark thoughts *and* cultivating more joy and well-being are the two reasons that meditation is so powerful. I urge you to begin these practices right away, starting with your post–Ganja Yoga time! Perhaps you take another toke before going into meditation, or perhaps you allow the high to dissipate as your body comes into a clear, meditative state. In either case, there are two final considerations to note before we get into the "Om Zone."

Comfort and Stillness

Pain and physical tension are some of the biggest obstacles to meditation. It's important to be as comfortable and as still as possible. Many beginners find this difficult, but it's just part of the practice. Use props so you're as supported as possible.

There is a healing quality to stillness that we rarely get the opportunity to cultivate. As you lie down for this practice, be sure the head, neck, and spine are aligned. Adjust your clothes and your body until you are completely comfortable. If the desire to move arises, see if you can just watch the desire. However, if there is discomfort or pain, make mindful movements to find maximum comfort.

Sometimes during meditation practice, we unconsciously adjust our posture out of boredom. Notice when you feel the urge to adjust your body. Is the movement enhancing or distracting your effort to enter the meditative state? Over time, you will be able to just *sit with* the urge and notice it without necessarily moving. Having said that, never, ever force your body to stay in a certain way, especially if you feel anything beyond minor discomfort.

We'll be covering two different types of meditations here: *embodiment* and *concentration*. For each, please read the description, and then when you get to the practice section, either read through it and then rely on your memory and intuition to guide you as you do the meditation or visit www.theganjayoga.com to get the audio for the guided meditations, read by yours truly.

Embodiment Meditation

Many of us don't notice the stiffness and soreness we hold in our body until we lie back and unwind with (or without) our pipe after a long day. When we finally let go and become present, we begin to feel just how much ache and tension we unconsciously carry in our day-to-day lives.

This also holds true for the mental and emotional tension we don't realize we're coping with. Things like bright lights, loud noises, emotionally draining people, strong fragrances, and tight clothing are microstressors of the nervous system, but we're often too distracted by business to notice them, let alone the stronger signals of distress our body tries to send us.

This meditation will help you come in touch with your body. Maybe you will find pain, maybe tightness, maybe relaxation. Embodiment meditation is the first step toward connecting to and releasing whatever does not work for your body. It's a great stand-alone practice or one that can be done after yogic movements of any kind.

THE PRACTICE

Lie on your back on your yoga mat or on a pile of folded blankets, a soft carpet, or the bed. Use a thin pillow or folded bath towel under the head and upper shoulder blades to undo some of the forward curve that most of us have in our spines. If the lower back feels tense, a small pillow under the knees can release tightness there.

You may also wish to cover yourself with a blanket. After yoga practice, our body temperature can significantly drop, so make sure you're nice and warm, so your muscles can relax completely. You may also wish to place something over your eyes to block out any additional light. Do whatever you need to do to feel as relaxed and supported as possible.

We're going to start by bringing the attention to each body part in sequence. As you bring your awareness to each part, take a moment to stretch, rotate, shake, or adjust joints or muscles near that part. Let's start by taking the awareness to the feet. Feel your feet, moving them as you'd like so they can be most relaxed. Now, feel the feet relax. Feel your lower legs; stretch, move, and relax the lower legs. Then let them rest on the floor. Next feel your knees and upper legs. Let them be relaxed. Feel your hips and buttocks, your pelvis and lower back, all as relaxed as can be. Feel your whole spine, your shoulder blades, and let these relax, adjusting as needed to release tension. Feel your belly and chest, moving as needed to be more comfortable and soft. Gently roll your head from side to side to allow the neck to relax, then return to center. Stretch your arms, then relax the upper and lower arms. Stretch and relax your hands. Squish up the muscles of your face and then let them relax.

Now come into Corpse Pose. Spread your legs slightly and let your feet drop open, so the lower back can be most relaxed. Open the arms away from the body, so the armpits are open and the shoulders can be most relaxed. Turn your palms up in a gesture of openness.

Once you're comfortable, try not to move. Feel your whole body relaxed, and see if you can remain still. Let your body sink into the floor. If pain or discomfort arises and you need to adjust your body, make your movement as small as you can. See if you can commit to stillness.

Put yourself in a mood to relax. Relax your cares, your personality, your entire being. Relax the mind, the intellect, the emotions. Feel a sense of cool water washing over your mind, cleansing it of concerns and distractions. Just be in your body. If your mind wanders to something that is not the sensations of the body, return the awareness, gently, promptly, continually—back to the body.

Discover a sense of equilibrium on the right and left sides. Just let your body relax as you feel the whole body on the floor. Allow yourself to rest here, softening the muscles, and channeling the cannabis high into your body. Using mindfulness, observe your body, allowing and accepting whatever arises. Your stomach gurgles. Your neck is tight. Your nose is itchy. Your belly moves when you breathe. Your blood flows. You feel a bit horny, a bit hot, a bit sore. Then let it go. Just keep noticing your body. Experience yourself in this moment.

If your mind begins to wander to thoughts and concerns, simply come back to the blissful experience of your body relaxing. As you keep noticing, the more you relax and soften. Even if you notice pain. Even if emotions arise. Just feel all seventy trillion of the cells in your body, inviting them to become more and more relaxed.

Focusing your attention on your body like this actually contributes to going beyond the body altogether in meditation, into inner experiences that cannot be described, only felt. The main purpose of meditation is to transcend the usual limitations of consciousness and permanently expand to higher levels of awareness. It begins with fully entering the body and giving it your full attention. We develop a body memory of bliss. It becomes our natural state, our baseline, for more and more profound inner experiences.

Nowhere else to be . . . Nothing else to do . . . This is your time . . . Stay with it . . . Feeling the body.

Our session is nearly complete. Feel the state of your body and mind as a result of your cannabis-enhanced embodiment meditation. Notice how you feel: your energy level, your mood, your body. Now become aware of your beating heart. Smile at your heart center. Feel love for your body, love for yourself.

And, without opening your eyes, start to have a sense of the room you are lying in. Visualize the ceiling, the floor, the four walls . . . and your body lying on the floor. See your whole body lying on the floor. Visualize the posture of your body, your clothing, even the expression on your face.

Now, as you take your next few breaths, allow your breathing to deepen. Begin to drink in the breath, letting it once more be deep and full. Feel your belly expand as you take in fresh life-force energy through the breath. And, as though inspired by the breathing, your fingers begin to slowly wake up and make movements. Your toes begin to wiggle, signaling to the body that meditation is now complete. As you continue to breathe deeply, rotate your wrists . . . your ankles . . . Take your time, stay relaxed.

AUTOSUGGESTION

After meditation practice and just before or just after sleep are said to be times when the subconscious aspects of the mind are most receptive to suggestions that can improve one's life. An autosuggestion is a short, concise sentence with clear, simple language that describes an intention you have. It should be positively worded and in the present tense. For example, instead of "I will be relaxed" (not present tense) or "I am free from stress" (not positively worded), a good sentence would be "I am relaxed."

When you mentally repeat your autosuggestion after meditation, let yourself have a feeling of its truth as you state it. The more gratitude and intensity you can bring into your autosuggestion, the more potency it will have.

As you emerge from this yoga practice, feel as though you've been bathed in a cool mountain stream, and know that this is a state of relaxation that you can come back to each and every time you practice.

Concentration Meditation

Unlike mindfulness, where the awareness is holistic, in concentration meditation we endeavor to keep the awareness on a specific object, such as the breath, a mantra, an image, a body part, or a sound.

This meditation practice will relieve the mind of mental congestion to reveal the clear sky of awareness behind. It will also slowly train the mind to become better at focusing. When our attention is scattered in many different directions, meditation becomes impossible. Concentration practices help us to focus our attention (even if we have an attention deficit), so over time we can begin to become aware of *awareness itself*. This takes us beyond the many thoughts that fragment the attention.

We all have the ability to cultivate better concentration, despite the bombardment by stimulation and distraction in our culture. Once you're able to focus the mind even a little bit, you can live life beyond the constant internal mental chatter; the mind begins to go beyond its normal scope, a vastness that can only be experienced.

According to yoga, the most important human goal is enlightenment. Enlightenment means full liberation from the illusion that you are separate from the rest of the universe, a total release from the egoic delusion that keeps you from realizing you are divine. According to yoga, meditation is the best way to attain this enlightened state of realization.

When we gently focus the mind on an object, such as the breath, a mantra, or a candle flame, the free-flowing impressions from the lower layers of mind can bubble up. Thoughts, visions, and memories (some deep-rooted) can come to the surface. Some of the content is random impressions, and some of it is unconscious parts of self that need to be worked through before full psychological and spiritual evolution can occur.

To work through anything dark that comes up during meditation, we simply allow the experience (thought, feeling, memory, or association). We bring full awareness to it; we do our best to accept it. Meditation helps us to become detached from thoughts and feelings, seeing them as *objects we can observe*, not as the *self*. In time, we're less impacted by any darker or more troubling thoughts and feelings we have, and we can fully release them, with no other "work" required but attention and acceptance.

When you realize you're no longer aware of your breath (or other object of meditation), come back it. Time and time again. Without emotion or attachment. That's the practice. Sometimes it will feel blissful; sometimes it will be boring. A quiet mind may result, perhaps there will be insights about the mental noise, or some days it may feel like a struggle. Staying diligent in the practice and noticing the contents of your mind as you do are what's important, not a particular outcome. In time, you will reach a deep calm, even if your day-to-day practice contains various experiences.

Decide what the *object* of your concentration will be. It could be a body part, a chakra, a candle flame, an image of a deity, the sun as it sets, a symbol, a tree, someone's eyes, a sound, a feeling, a mantra, a word, the breath, or your sparkly new bong. Whatever you choose, you keep your mind focused on it (and your eyes too, if it's a visual object).

For the purpose of this meditation, we will remain focused on the breath. It is always with us, so it's an easy object for beginners to start with. Allow the cannabis to deepen both your connection to your body as it relaxes here, and the depth of your breathing, which is effortless and relaxed. Whenever the mind wanders, simply return to the breath and the body. This practice can be done in any position. Wiggle your body so you feel comfortable, balanced on the right and left sides, and relaxed. Continue to adjust very subtly whenever you feel uncomfortable, finding as much stillness as you can throughout the meditation. The more relaxed and still your body is, the more relaxed and still your mind will be.

Again, either you can read through this and then let memory and intuition guide you in your meditation, or you can get the guided audio at www.theganjayoga.com.

THE PRACTICE

To begin, take a deep breath, and as you breathe out, feel the cares and worries of your day floating out of you. Repeat twice, and with each long exhalation, release distractions, anxieties, and concerns from your mind and body.

Now let the deep breathing go, and simply watch the breath, letting it be natural and effortless. You might silently repeat the phrase "I am breathing in," each time you inhale, and "I am breathing out" each time you release the breath.

Let the awareness clearly illuminate the sensation of breathing in the body, either at the belly or the nostrils. Let the mind flow as it does.

Do not let a single breath come in or go out without gently concentrating on it. How can you make the breath the most fascinating thing for your awareness to discover? What can you notice about it? Where do you feel it moving your body, naturally, effortlessly? How does it feel to breathe, to be—right here, right now?

Feel the movement of the belly gently rising and falling with the breath, without doing anything to consciously change it. As you allow the body to breathe, noticing each inhalation and each exhalation, you are becoming more and more relaxed in your body and in your mind.

Continue to watch each breath, but know that concentration practices should not cause strain or tension. We're not looking for a contracted, sharp, laser beam of attention here. In meditation, a degree of effort is involved, but it shouldn't be strenuous. It's steady and constant, like a flame in a windless room.

Cultivate relaxed focus. Even though we're focusing the mind, meditation practice should be as effortless as possible.

Just watch the breath and be, repeating the mantra "I am breathing in" and "I am breathing out," if you'd like.

What comes up for you as you do this? Merge into the present moment. If there's an ache in your body or a noise outside, let your awareness be with it, notice it, let your meditation include it instead of letting it feel like a distraction from your meditation.

This is especially true for thoughts in your mind. At first, they may seem relentless. But the more you give them permission to exist, the less distracting the thoughts will be. Don't worry about the thoughts; just keep your awareness steady on your breath. Think of your mind as a puppy that you are gently training. Our culture has conditioned it to go off into thoughts. You're giving it a new challenge, so be patient with it as it learns to stay focused on one thing.

WHERE TO WATCH THE BREATH

Focusing the attention on the breath at the belly tends to decrease mental activity and helps in feeling more connected to the body and blissful. Focusing on the breath at the nostrils tends to bring clarity of awareness and transcendent experiences. Over the course of several meditation practices, try both a few times, and see what the difference is for you.

You are just watching the breath. Whenever you notice that the mind has pulled your awareness away from the feeling of the body relaxing and the feeling of your breath, practice the art of softly, gently, lovingly, and patiently guiding the awareness back to the breathing, keeping the body totally relaxed.

Bring the awareness to the softening of the belly, while also keeping the awareness on the breath. Feel the belly breathe. Notice each inhalation and each exhalation. By now the breathing should be totally effortless. Keep it in the belly; just let it naturally soften so there's no "doing," only watching. There is nowhere else to be, nothing else to do. Just breathe. Just watch.

Instead of "trying to relax" in meditation, use meditation to see things as they are. If there's pain, see it. Invite relaxation, but if that isn't possible, just be with what is. Continue to watch your breath rise and fall in your belly. Continue to feel your whole body relaxing. The more we bring awareness and acceptance to our habitual mental reactions, things like boredom, discomfort, pain, and judgment, the less struggle and suffering we usually experience.

The ability to focus the mind is something that we can all strengthen. Remember, it isn't about trying to clear the mind. Meditation practice is about noticing your mind as you remain diligently and relaxedly aware of your breath. You do not have to make the mind calm; you simply have to observe the fluctuations of the mind, and they'll quiet on their own.

Stay in this practice as long as you like. When you're ready to release, let go of the practice of concentrating the attention and just relax. Feel yourself quiet, peaceful, and tranquil, while at the same time revived and refreshed. Spend some time being quiet after meditation, just enjoying the fruits of your practice.

MEDITATION TIPS

- According to yoga, the best times to meditate are early morning and at night before bed. Choose a time that is most convenient for you, so you're more likely to stick with it. (Did somebody say wake 'n' bake?!)

- The duration is up to you. Some people use a timer and others end when it feels right. Start with five to ten minutes and work up from there.

- You can meditate sitting, lying down, standing, walking, or in any yoga pose. I recommend the Corpse Pose, with a pillow under the head and tops of shoulders.

- If you frequently find yourself falling asleep during meditation, splash cold water on your face or place a cool damp cloth at the back of the neck just before practicing. If this doesn't help, meditate seated so you'll be less drowsy. Or skip meditation and go to bed.

- If you're more tired after meditation than you are energized, it might mean you're fighting with your mind or concentrating too hard. Aim to be relaxed and aware.

- Release any judgment about whether you are doing the practice correctly. That's just more mind. Be compassionate with your wandering mind.

- Repeat an autosuggestion after meditation to plant seeds for healing and growth. Some examples: "I am healthy and strong," "I am relaxed and confident," "I feel grateful and positive."

- Massage the scalp after meditation to remove congestion and allow the energies of well-being to flow.

- The most important piece of advice I can give you is to be consistent and dedicated. The insights, relaxation, and blissful experiences affect you for days after you meditate, and you continue to grow the more you practice.

The Gift That Keeps on Giving

Meditation works by slowly freeing your mind of the mental programs you unconsciously run. As you learn to see your thoughts and release them, you're able to let other things go. Ego-based conflict that used to rile you up and cause you stress becomes water off a duck's back. The restorative movements and mindful yoga poses you do rebalance your adrenal glands and other hormonal secretions. Your muscles, bones, and connective tissues get the forces they need to be strong and healthy. Deep yogic breathing feeds your body and brings more energy and relaxation to body and mind.

Cannabis, nature's wonder drug, stimulates your body's innate ability to self-heal naturally.

Each of these is extraordinary on its own, but when they're all combined, unimaginable levels of happiness and health can be attained.

Your pain, your level of happiness, your connection to others, your health, your creativity, your childlike joy, and so many other aspects of your life can be enhanced with intentional breathing and moving and educated, conscious cannabis use.

The Divine Stoner in me sees the Divine Stoner in you.

Namaste.

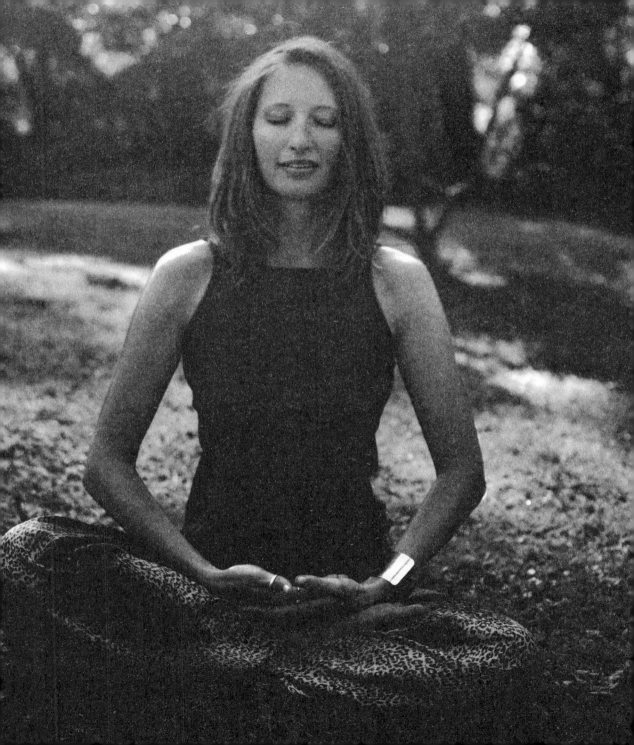

CONCLUSION:
BETTER LIVING THROUGH CHEMISTRY

Cannabis and yoga are two of the best technologies our species has to help us thrive, despite what is at the moment a pathological civilization. "Life, liberty, and the pursuit of happiness" is the birthright of every American, yet we aren't encouraged to exercise the freedom to do as we wish with our body chemistry and state of consciousness. In fact, we have been punished.

This is finally changing. As legalization gains momentum, normalization spreads like a weed. As culture makes room for the bikini babes with their bongs, the hip-hop stars with their 24k gold rolling papers, and the CBD medications for the kids with seizures, we have a unique opportunity to *normalize cannabis use for every person who wants to integrate it as part of a holistic approach to health.*

By using cannabis intentionally, alongside either various yoga practices or other consciousness-awakening activities like journaling, expressive art, dancing, therapy, and time with nature, your awareness *will* start to transform, and with it the aspects of your personality that no longer serve you. This purification is one of the aims of yoga. Slowly but surely, internalized habits and unconscious patterns begin to surface, and with awareness and acceptance they slowly get released.

In place of the defense mechanisms, pettiness, scarcity, distrust, and the desire to control others, we tap into a wellspring of energy and capacity for love. We care less about material success, what others think, egoic identifications, and superficial concerns. This doesn't mean we become ascetic. Rather, we become caretakers of our possessions and each other and champions of justice for all.

Yoga posits that there is a vast terrain of unexplored abilities to be discovered as we actualize our potential. Although the practice of yoga brings countless benefits, the most important is that it reminds us of the significance of existence. We don't need to change our lifestyle, thoughts, identifications, or desires; we just do the practices and see if we become better people.

Even a little effort toward cultivating mindfulness and relaxation brings incredible returns in energy and harmonious interpersonal relationships. You won't know until you try. Remember, yoga values scientific exploration, and you are both the scientist and the laboratory. Yoga practice is about taking yourself off autopilot and becoming more embodied and wise, enjoying more harmony with others and a more relaxed outlook on and experience of life.

Ganja Yoga redefines yoga, not because practitioners are stoned, but because it removes its current fitness orientation and instead *prioritizes it for relaxation, personal development, and spiritual evolution.*

Pot Progress and Cannabis Culture

Remember this: cannabis has been used medicinally for *thousands of years*. This should *not* be cutting-edge, controversial medicine. But it is, because most doctors the world over still remain completely ignorant of the endocannabinoid system, despite the fact it is a *central component* of health.

Our democratically elected officials lied to us about cannabis. Antimarijuana campaigns funded by large corporations went hand in hand with racism against Mexican and African Americans. Myths about the harms of cannabis have benefitted pharmaceutical, alcohol, prison, and tobacco companies, which spend a lot of money lobbying against legalization. Things are improving, but they do take time.

After having an awakening to "cannabis consciousness," it's natural to want to share all of this with others. It's understandable to want to shout it from the rooftops! But be patient as you share new information with reluctant loved ones. We are just waking up from a *century* of mass conditioning about the "evils of marijuana," and we each have our own pace as we lift the curtain.

As we calmly educate others about the scientifically proven benefits, we affect public perception, which affects policy and government decision, which helps reform laws that keep so many of our brothers and sisters, es-

> "We have been terribly and systematically misled for nearly seventy years in the United States, and I apologize for my own role in that."
> —Dr. Sanjay Gupta, Chief Medical Correspondent, CNN

pecially people of color, needlessly suffering in prisons. By coming out of the cannabis closet, we give others the permission to do the same, bringing more information and building community, helping to ensure safe and affordable access for all. If we can get safe and affordable access for everyone, this single plant could positively impact the health of nearly everyone on earth.

In the meantime, half of the states allow medical cannabis use, and a handful have made adult use fully legal. Canada and Jamaica just legalized, and Mexico may be following suit. Not to mention Amsterdam and Uruguay.

It's clear that the future belongs to us.

That's right, *us*. You are a part of this unfolding, this global awakening. I don't know how you got here, what brought you to yoga or weed, what strains you like, or what poses calm you down. But we're buds now, you and I, along with the tens of thousands of others out there like us.

I don't like to share this, but *no one* showed up to my first Ganja Yoga class. *Not one person*. I almost cried and texted my friend with the bummer news, but instead I got high and did my practice. I set up the candles and rolled such a good doobie, it would have been a waste not to. Sure, no one came, but I believed in the practice, even if it was a party of one.

But now you're here.

Let's get started.

APPENDIX I:
The New "Green Smoothie"

Cannabis improves the function of your immune system, reduces inflammation, and fights pain, anxiety, depression, and insomnia, while improving neural function, bone growth, and metabolism. Not to mention, it kills cancer. Cannabis is truly the most important vegetable on the planet. Okay, I might be biased, but I think we can all agree it's more fun than kale.

Just like other greens, though, juicing raw cannabis leaves takes this dietary supplement to the next level. The body can tolerate far more cannabinoids when they are consumed in their raw form. Think about the antioxidant and neuroprotective benefits that occur when you take hundreds or even thousands of milligrams of cannabidiolic acid (CBDA) and tetrahydrocannabinolic acid (THCA) instead of just a few dozen milligrams of CBD and THC from edibles, vapes, smoking, or dabs. Kind of like those green smoothies that pack pounds of veggies into one glass.

In order for raw weed to be turned into something that will get you high, it must be decarboxylated (heated to 200 degrees Fahrenheit), which converts it into THC. (This is why this smoothie won't get you high, but you'll still reap the benefits of the herb.)

222

By consuming THCA, the acidic precursor to THC, found in freshly harvested buds, you'll get less of a psychoactive effect and more a sense of heightened well-being. It also has anti-inflammatory, antitumor, and antispasmodic compounds.

Remember, just because the leaves and raw buds aren't psychoactive, that doesn't mean the therapeutic effects of cannabinoids aren't huge!

DIRECTIONS

1. Be sure your juicer produces "cold pressed" juice, so no nutrients are lost. Make sure you have raw (uncured) organic cannabis. Have it cut up to fit into your juicer attachment.

2. Juice other fruits and vegetables for health and taste. Then add five to twenty cannabis leaves and, if possible, one or two raw buds. (Minimize the amount of fruit or other sugars to keep it as anti-inflammatory as possible.)

3. Drink and enjoy!

APPENDIX II:
The Ancient Ganja Milkshake

Bhang lassi, or "ganja milkshake," has been an important part of Hindu culture for at least three thousand years. Containing cannabis that was grown in the Himalayas (but thought to come from the gods), this sweet, spicy edible is consumed to deepen meditation. It is the yogic version of the Communion wafer, a sacrament for Lord Shiva. It is also used in Ayurvedic medicine. In Indian culture, spirituality and health are inextricably linked.

Traditionally, cannabis flower is cooked in warm cow's milk and then pounded in a mortar several times. In this version, my husband and I decarboxylated the cannabis to increase the psychoactive effect.

INGREDIENTS

- ¼ to ½ ounce cannabis, depending on desired potency
- 1 tablespoon melted butter (we use ghee to make it lactose-free; you could use coconut oil to make it vegan)
- 3 cups of milk, or milk alternative
- 2 tablespoons ground almonds or pistachios
- 8 whole cardamom pods, split and pounded in a mortar with a pestle to remove shells and break up seeds
- 1 teaspoon rose water

½ cup sugar (or ¼ cup honey plus ¼ cup maple syrup, to make it lower-glycemic)

OPTIONAL ADDITIONS

Rose petals

Mint leaves

¼ teaspoon any of the following: ginger (dried or fresh), fennel, anise, cinnamon, coriander seed, nutmeg, turmeric, vanilla bean

Matcha green tea powder, for garnish

DIRECTIONS

1. Decarb the cannabis: Preheat the oven to 240 degrees F. (115 degrees C.). Place the coarsely ground flower on a baking tray in a single layer. Make sure there is no empty space showing on the tray; if so, use a smaller tray. Toast for 30 to 40 minutes, stirring every 10 minutes.

2. Warm ½ cup of the milk and melt in the ghee. Grind small amounts of the decarboxylated cannabis with some of the warmed milk and ghee in a mortar with a pestle to extract it.

3. Add the almonds or pistachios and more warm milk as needed.

4. Strain, then add the remaining ingredients to the mix and blend.

5. Serve over ice, add garnish, and enjoy. (Serves 8.)

OM NAMAH SHIVAYA.

APPENDIX III:

More Ways to Enhance Your Endocannabinoid System

The endocannabinoid system (ECS) is an animal's way to adapt to environmental stressors. Since human lives are far more stressful than those of any other animals, we have to consciously take care of our endocannabinoid system to ensure it doesn't become depleted. Here are some ways to keep it functioning well that do not involve cannabis:

- Avoid stressful stimuli that deplete your endocannabinoid system.

- Cultivate mindful movement, breathing, and stillness (yoga), so your system is more resilient and doesn't have to work so hard.

- Do not eat inflammation-causing foods that tax your ECS. These include sugar, refined grains, trans fats, and the vegetable oils in most processed foods (canola, corn, soybean, margarine, shortening).

- Increase your intake of foods with essential omega-3 and omega-6 fatty acids, which are precursors for endocannabinoids. Mostly we need more of the omega-3s, since we get enough omega-6 in our vegetable oils. Eat from a range of the following foods to ensure you're getting all three types of omega-3 *fatties*!

- **hemp seeds**
- **flax seeds (and/or oil)**
- **omega-3-enhanced eggs**
- **sardines, salmon**
- **fish oil**
- **Brussels sprouts**
- **kale**
- **spinach**
- **cauliflower**
- **walnuts**
- **pumpkin seeds**
- **soybeans, tofu**
- **beef**
- **shrimp**

- Eat only the healthy omega-6 foods, like coconut oil, macadamia nut oil, sunflower oil, olive oil, wheat germ, walnut oil, sesame oil, and flaxseed oil.

- *Lactobacillus acidophilus* (a probiotic) induces endocannabinoid receptors in the intestines that provide analgesic effects similar to morphine.

- Other medical herbs, such as *Echinacea purpurea,* have been found to contain nonpsychoactive cannabinoids.

- Exercise greatly increases the production of anandamide, the body's naturally occurring cannabinoid.

APPENDIX IV:

Other Scientifically Proven Ways to Improve Your Health

Ganja Yoga is only one piece of the puzzle. Other things that benefit health are:

- **Movement.** As many muscles, joints, and bones, in as many ways, as often as you can!

- **Sunshine.** At least twenty minutes of outdoor time every day, more when the sun isn't shining.

- **Enough sleep.** Do whatever it takes to make it happen.

- **Protein.** More than you think, and more in the early part of the day.

- **Consensual, friendly touch.** Hugs, massages, cuddles. Even casual arm pats. Get more.

- **Sensual aliveness.** Sex, pleasure, masturbation, delicious food. We are organisms uniquely suited to enjoy a range of rewarding experiences. Why not do our best to ensure we have them?

- **Relaxation.** Every day we must unwind. Sleep is not the place for this. Relaxation has to be conscious.

- **Mindfulness.** Presence. There's nowhere else to be.

- **Doing something that doesn't benefit you personally.** It works. In India this is called Karma Yoga, or the yoga of selfless action. Pay it forward. You'll feel happier and make the world a better place.

- **Letting yourself feel and express emotion.** Journal, talk, cry, paint, dance, get a massage, howl, sigh. We are animals, not robots.

- **Nature, universal mother.** Reduce screen time and instead enjoy the birds, trees, and other creatures we share home with.

APPENDIX V:

Addressing Some Critiques of Enhanced Yoga

In case anyone wants to debate with you about whether your Ganja Yoga practice is a good idea, here are some frequently made criticisms and my responses.

THE EXPERIENCE IS NOT "REAL."

The "artificial paradise" argument is a common critique when it comes to using substances for spiritual purposes. It assumes the experiences had during a cannabis-enhanced yoga class are more superficial, transient, or illusory than those experienced sober. This basic assumption is entirely culturally conditioned and an outcome of our puritanical past. To insist on the "reality" of one form of conscious experience over others is to fundamentally misunderstand consciousness itself. It's all real, or perhaps it's more accurate to say that it is all illusion, a construct of your own subjective psyche.

It makes sense that people who put a lot of their time into their spiritual practices wouldn't like the idea of others being able to get to the same states of consciousness without devoting as much time. However, thousands of shamans from time immemorial, from every continent around the world, would certainly say these experiences are real.

GANJA YOGA IS SPIRITUAL "CHEATING."

Others accept that the spiritual experiences had on cannabis are real and meaningful, but accuse the ganja yogi of cheating the system to get there. Cannabis reduces our anxieties, soothes our muscle tension, fosters creativity and insight, and makes it easy to focus on sensations, making our yoga practice "too easy." In a capitalist economy as unequal as our own, free time for years of spiritual growth is a privilege of the rich. Yet we are all entitled to the pursuit. In my opinion, anything that shaves off surface tension so I can connect deeper to myself in my practice is an efficient use of time, not spiritual bypass. This "no pain, no gain" mentality makes little sense considering we're all on completely unique spiritual paths, and there is no race to the finish line.

YOGA DOESN'T NEED TO BE "ENHANCED."

Some people argue that we shouldn't *need* to use an external substance to enhance the perfect, whole, and complete practice of yoga. However, these very people think nothing of consuming mind-altering substances like chocolate or tea before practice. Nary a practitioner thinks twice about lighting candles or playing music to enhance a meditation or using breathing practices that have profound effects on our consciousness. Anyone who has sung Kirtan will tell you that the repetition and act of harmonizing changes consciousness. To insist that some of these are okay and others aren't is a false dichotomy.

Ancient yogis practiced on the bare floor. The really ancient ones practiced in caves. Yet there is no debate about enhancing with a cushy, store-bought mat.

As we know by now, the ideologies, practices, and beliefs of yoga have changed numerous times over the ages, and different yogic scriptures often contradict each other. As such, there is no one traditional or "correct" yoga. The authority is you. You can wear special yoga socks to keep you from slipping, use blocks to help you reach the floor, find peaceful music to take you deeper, and puff ganja if you want to. Almost all yoga is enhanced by something.

CANNABIS WILL OPEN "FALSE CHANNELS."

Some yogis claim cannabis and psychedelics leave negative energy consequences, creating false lines of energy in the physical body (organs, vessels, nerves, lymph) and the energy body (as treated in acupuncture). My yoga teacher told me this when I shared with her that the more I used cannabis, the more my practice was progressing. A tantric practitioner, she said to make sure it's *mindful use,* as it's been said that "false channels" cause us to lose our ability to relate to consensus reality and contribute to the world.

Whether or not you believe in energy channels, chakras, and meridians, the response here is to be mindful. If you feel as though you're losing touch with the "default world" from too much Ganja Yoga, come on back to us. Make sure you're still meeting your responsibilities and taking pleasure in a range of things.

A TOOL CAN BECOME A CRUTCH.

This critique is perhaps the one I have spent the most time pondering myself. I've heard concern from many people about coming to *rely on* cannabis for relaxation and transformation, and when I started my journey, I was aware of not wanting to fall into the trap of addiction, having dealt with opioid addiction in my family when I was a teenager.

I kept telling myself things like, "Okay, I am going to consume only *three times* this week" (or, after I moved to the West Coast, "only three times *today*"), setting parameters to prevent dependence. At the same time, it didn't feel completely right to be treating cannabis like alcohol or a party drug, especially the more I came to understand its enormous medical and spiritual power.

Any tool can become a crutch if we're not mindful of it. If we reach for our yoga block day in and day out without ever seeing if we can do the pose without it, we may hinder the development of our practice. If we come to need soft music to really relax, the organized calm of a retreat center, or, yes, a little hoot from the pipe, then our spiritual practice may have a gap that we could bring awareness to. Because what if there's no block, soft music, or weed? Are you going to be able to deal?

The first step is to notice when a reliance or habit of any kind is starting to form, without judgment or emotion. The second step is to cul-

LIVE AND LET LIVE

People can enhance their practice if they're called to, in any way they're called to. This includes using various perfumed incenses, drinking a cacao smoothie before class, or meditating in the sun. These are all ways to change consciousness, and it is our right to do just that. Some people may not be called to use ganja—on a particular day, during a particular phase of their life, or over the course of their whole life, and that's totally dandy.

tivate the discipline needed to sometimes do something else, for balance. If music is turning from "tool" to "crutch" for you, be sure to do a few yoga sessions without your trippy beats. If you find you're getting reliant on retreat environments to keep your cool, see if you can do your best to find mindfulness on a noisy bus.

All medicine becomes a poison at the wrong dose. Be present to your relationship with cannabis and find the frequency and dose that support you the best. Not all habits are deleterious, so use self-awareness to help you decide if your cannabis use is serving you, and take breaks every now and again if it feels useful.

CANNABIS WILL SPOIL US.

Another fear is that using cannabis regularly will make us less appreciative of sober existence. All of the beautiful little gifts of grace the universe throws our way every moment of every day will be ignored, and we'll only be able to "tap in" spiritually when we're high.

Obviously as a spiritual practitioner, I encourage you to be present, appreciative, and connected to yourself and the divine or cosmos or whatever you call it, every moment you can—stoned or sober.

Despite the fact that I have been supplementing with cannabis for years, I've never had a problem feeling happy, appreciative, and joyful about life when I need to be sober (like visiting a foreign country or in-laws). If you happen to not have cannabis on that hike or at that great restaurant or before making out with that new person, well, it's not a big deal. If it *is* a big deal, you may have a dependency (if so, go back to Chapter 11).

Bottom line: cannabis is a modulator, a life-enhancer.

A happy life is lived with awareness and a sense of balance in all aspects.

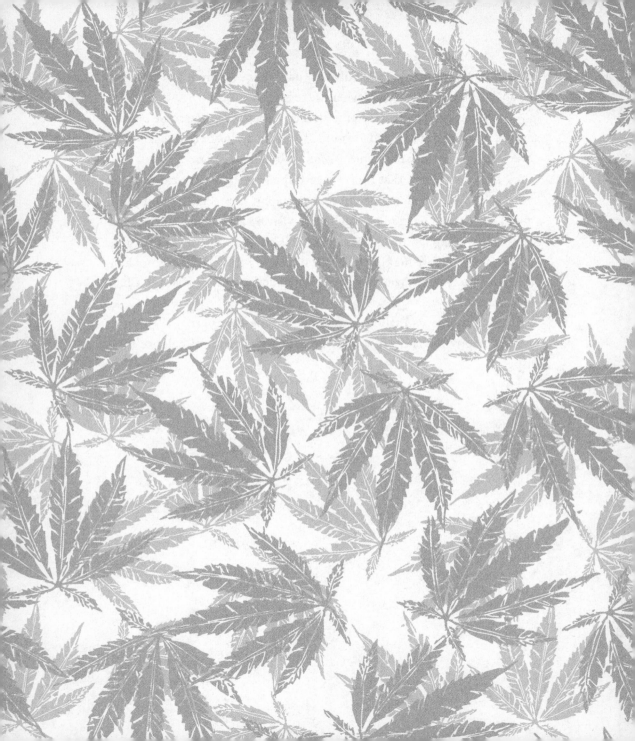

FURTHER READING

ALIGNMENT MATTERS, by Katy Bowman

ASANA PRANAYAMA MUDRA BANDHA,
by Swami Satyananda Saraswati

CANNABIS AND SPIRITUALITY, edited by Stephen Gray

CANNABIS AND THE SOMA SOLUTION, by Chris Bennett

THE CANNABIS MANIFESTO, by Steve DeAngelo

**CANNABIS IN MEDICAL PRACTICE: A LEGAL, HISTORICAL, AND
PHARMACOLOGICAL OVERVIEW OF THE THERAPEUTIC USE OF
MARIJUANA,** by Mary Lynn Mathre

HOW TO SMOKE POT (PROPERLY), by David Bienenstock

MEDITATIONS FROM THE TANTRAS, by Swami Satyananda Saraswati

MOVE YOUR DNA, by Katy Bowman

STRETCH: THE UNLIKELY MAKING OF A YOGA DUDE,
by Neal Pollack

YOGA 2.0, by Matthew Remski and Scott Petrie

THE YOGA OF MARIJUANA, by Joan Bello

YOGA NIDRA, by Swami Satyananda Saraswati

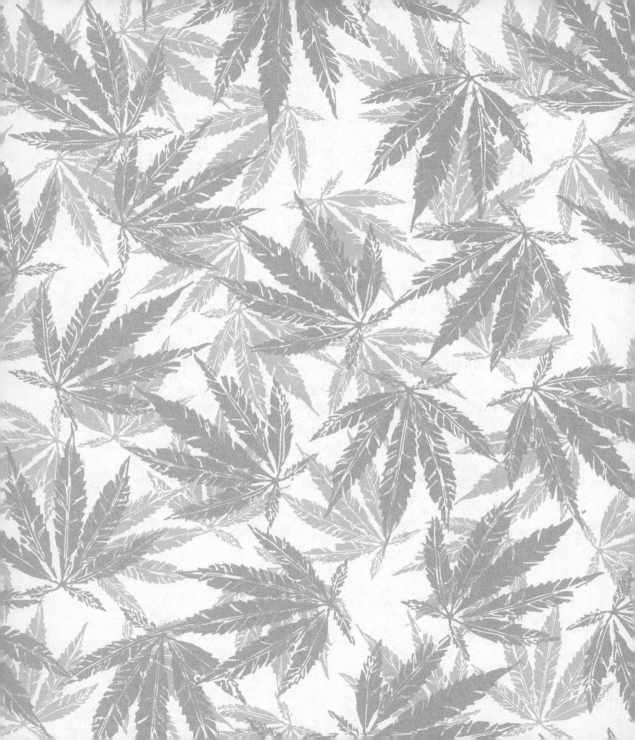

ACKNOWLEDGMENTS

First, gratitude to the herb for taking my yoga to the next level.

Thank you, Allie Butler, for turning me on to dabs and for providing good medicine to people. Thanks as well to my editor, Hilary Lawson, for all your hard work and good ideas, and to our whole HarperCollins team: Ann Moru, Sydney Rogers, Nadea Mina, Lisa Zuniga, and Ann Edwards. Incredible gratitude to Ali Pinkerton, my feminist high school gym teacher, and the first person to show me what it could be like to live a rich and meaningful life.

Thank you to my teacher, Ananda Shakti, from Toronto, and her teacher, Swami Satyananda Saraswati, from Bihar, India, for making esoteric tantric yoga teachings available to anyone. Thank you, biochemist Katy Bowman, for making body science easy to understand. You saved my back!

Thank you to every student who inspired my work and reconfirmed the need for these teachings. Thanks as well to my mom for buying me that random yoga DVD in 1995. You changed my world.

Most of all, thank you to my husband, Scott Finnell. Your creative insights, brilliant editing suggestions, and tireless fact-checking breathed air into this baby. Thank you for your expertise on the history chapter, for the exquisite meals and great sex, and for keeping my pipe filled throughout. I couldn't have done this without you. XO.

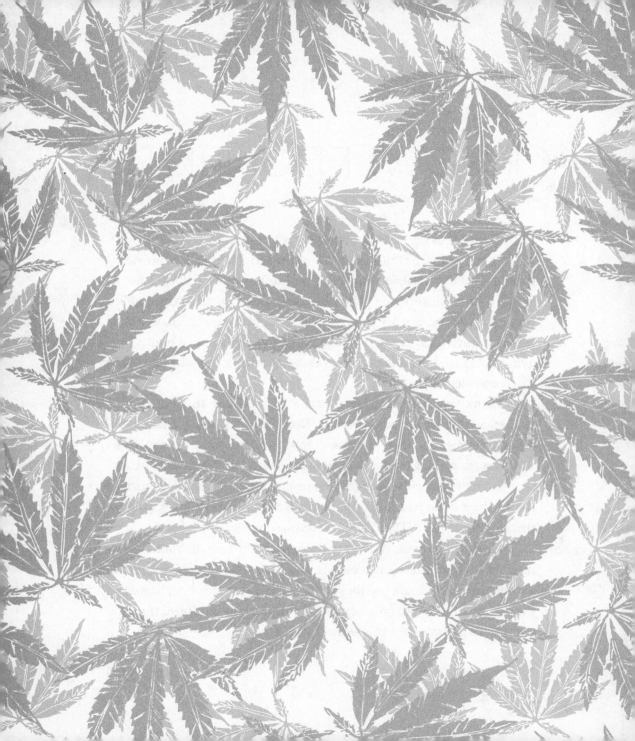

REFERENCES

CHAPTER 1: CANNABIS AS MEDICINE

Ali, S. F., G. D. Newport, A. C. Scallet, M. G. Paule, J. R. Bailey, and W. Slikker. November 1991. "Chronic marijuana smoke exposure in the rhesus monkey. IV: Neurochemical effects and comparison to acute and chronic exposure to delta-9-tetrahydrocannabinol (THC) in rats." *Pharmacology, Biochemistry, and Behavior* 40 (3): 677–82.

American Psychological Association. "How stress affects your health." http://www.apa.org/helpcenter/stress.aspx.

Armentano, Paul. August 28, 2015. "Recent research on medical marijuana." *NORML,* http://norml.org/component/zoo/category/recent-research-on-medical-marijuana.

Bergamaschi, Mateus Machado, Regina Helena Costa Queiroz, Antonio Waldo Zuardi, and José Alexandre S. Crippa. September 2, 2011. "Safety and side effects of cannabidiol, a cannabis sativa constituent." *Current Drug Safety* 6 (4): 237–49.

Beulaygue, Isabelle C., and Michael T. French. September 2016. "Got munchies? Estimating the relationship between marijuana use and body mass index." *Journal of Mental Health Policy and Economics* 19 (3): 123–40.

Bluett, R. J., J. C. Gamble-George, D. J. Hermanson, N. D. Hartley, L. J. Marnett, and S. Patel. 2014. "Central anandamide deficiency predicts stress-induced

anxiety: Behavioral reversal through endocannabinoid augmentation."
Translational Psychiatry 4: e408, doi:10.1038/tp.2014.53.

Cheng, David, Adena S. Spiro, Andrew M. Jenner, Brett Garner, and Tim Karl. 2014. "Long-term cannabidiol treatment prevents the development of social recognition memory deficits in Alzheimer's Disease transgenic mice." *Journal of Alzheimer's Disease* 42 (4): 1383–96, doi:10.3233/JAD-140921.

Consroe, P., and A. Wolkin. April 1977. "Cannabidiol—antiepileptic drug comparisons and interactions in experimentally induced seizures in rats." *Journal of Pharmacology and Experimental Therapeutics* 201 (1): 26–32.

de Filippis, Daniele, Giuseppe Esposito, Carla Cirillo, Mariateresa Cipriano, Benedicte Y. De Winter, Caterina Scuderi, Giovanni Sarnelli, Rosario Cuomo, Luca Steardo, Joris G. De Man, and Teresa Iuvone. 2011. "Cannabidiol reduces intestinal inflammation through the control of neuroimmune axis." *PloS One* 6 (12): e28159, doi:10.1371/journal.pone.0028159.

de Mello Schier, Alexandre R., Natalia P. de Oliveira Ribeiro, Danielle S. Coutinho, Sergio Machado, Oscar Arias-Carrión, Jose A. Crippa, Antonio W. Zuardi, Antonio E. Nardi, and Adriana C. Silva. 2014. "Antidepressant-like and anxiolytic-like effects of cannabidiol: A chemical compound of cannabis sativa." *CNS & Neurological Disorders—Drug Targets* 13 (6): 953–60.

Dohenny, Kathleen. August 30, 2010. "Marijuana relieves chronic pain, research shows." *WebMD,* http://www.webmd.com/pain-management/news/20100830/marijuana-relieves-chronic-pain-research-show.

Doyle, Kathryn. August 25, 2014. "Prescription painkiller deaths fall in medical marijuana states." http://news.yahoo.com/prescription-painkiller-deaths-fall-medical-marijuana-states-202837041.html?ref=gs.

Fields, R. Douglas. 2007. "Sex and the secret nerve." *Scientific American Mind* 18 (1): 20–27, doi:10.1038/scientificamericanmind0207–20.

Fiz, Jimena, Marta Durán, Dolors Capellà, Jordi Carbonell, and Magí Farré. 2011. "Cannabis use in patients with fibromyalgia: Effect on symptoms relief and health-related quality of life." *PloS One* 6 (4): e18440, doi:10.1371/journal .pone.0018440.

Fuller, G. N., and P. C. Burger. December 1990. "Nervus terminalis (cranial nerve zero) in the adult human." *Clinical Neuropathology* 9 (6): 279–83.

Gonzalez, Robbie. July 29, 2014. "How a mysterious body part called fascia is challenging medicine." *io9.gizmodo,* http://io9.gizmodo.com/how-a-mysterious-body-part-called-fascia-is-challenging-1598939224.

Gupta, Sanjay. March 11, 2014. "Medical marijuana and the 'entourage effect.'" *CNN,* http://www.cnn.com/2014/03/11/health/gupta-marijuana-entourage/index.html.

Hampson, A. J., M. Grimaldi, J. Axelrod, and D. Wink. July 7, 1998. "Cannabidiol and (–)Δ9-tetrahydrocannabinol are neuroprotective antioxidants." *Proceedings of the National Academy of Sciences* 95 (14): 8268–73.

Hampson, A. J., M. Grimaldi, M. Lolic, D. Wink, R. Rosenthal, and J. Axelrod. 2000. "Neuroprotective antioxidants from marijuana." *Annals of the New York Academy of Sciences* 899: 274–82.

Hartley, J. P., S. G. Nogrady, and A. Seaton. June 1978. "Bronchodilator effect of delta1-tetrahydrocannabinol." *British Journal of Clinical Pharmacology* 5 (6): 523–25.

Hill, Matthew N., and Boris B. Gorzalka. September 2005. "Is there a role for the endocannabinoid system in the etiology and treatment of melancholic depression?" *Behavioral Pharmacology* 16 (5–6): 333–52.

———. December 1, 2009. "The endocannabinoid system and the treatment of mood and anxiety disorders." *CNS & Neurological Disorders—Drug Targets* (formerly *Current Drug Targets*) 8 (6): 451–58, doi:10.2174/187152709789824624.

Iuvone, Teresa, Giuseppe Esposito, Ramona Esposito, Rita Santamaria, Massimo Di Rosa, and Angelo A. Izzo. April 2004. "Neuroprotective effect of cannabidiol, a non-psychoactive component from cannabis sativa, on beta-amyloid-induced toxicity in pc12 cells." *Journal of Neurochemistry* 89 (1): 134–41, doi:10.1111/j.1471–4159.2003.02327.x.

Malfait, A. M., R. Gallily, P. F. Sumariwalla, A. S. Malik, E. Andreakos, R. Mechoulam, and M. Feldmann. August 15, 2000. "The nonpsychoactive cannabis constituent cannabidiol is an oral anti-arthritic therapeutic in murine collagen-induced arthritis." *Proceedings of the National Academy of Sciences of the USA* 97 (17): 9561–66, doi:10.1073/pnas.160105897.

Manchikanti, Laxmaiah, Standiford Helm, Bert Fellows, Jeffrey W. Janata, Vidyasagar Pampati, Jay S. Grider, and Mark V. Boswell. July 2012. "Opioid epidemic in the United States." *Pain Physician* 15 (3 Suppl): ES9–38.

Miller, Kelli. April 1, 2009. "Marijuana chemical may fight brain cancer." *WebMD*, http://www.webmd.com/cancer/brain-cancer/news/20090401/marijuana-chemical-may-fight-brain-cancer.

Nagarkatti, Prakash, Rupal Pandey, Sadiye Amcaoglu Rieder, Venkatesh L. Hegde, and Mitzi Nagarkatti. October 2009. "Cannabinoids as novel anti-inflammatory drugs." *Future Medicinal Chemistry* 1 (7): 1333–49, doi:10.4155/fmc.09.93.

NORML. July 16, 2015. "Study: Medical Cannabis Access Associated with Reduced Opioid Abuse." http://norml.org/news/2015/07/16/study-medical-cannabis-access-associated-with-reduced-opioid-abuse.

Passie, Torsten, Hinderk M. Emrich, Matthias Karst, Simon D. Brandt, and John H. Halpern. July 1, 2012. "Mitigation of post-traumatic stress symptoms by cannabis resin: A review of the clinical and neurobiological evidence." *Drug Testing and Analysis* 4 (7–8): 649–59, doi:10.1002/dta.1377.

Penner, Elizabeth A., Hannah Buettner, and Murray A. Mittleman. July 2013. "The impact of marijuana use on glucose, insulin, and insulin resistance among US adults." *American Journal of Medicine* 126 (7): 583–89, doi:10.1016/j.amjmed.2013.03.002

Preidt, Robert. April 13, 2015. "Liquid medical marijuana shows promise against severe epilepsy." *WebMD*, http://www.webmd.com/epilepsy/news/20150413/liquid-medical-marijuana-shows-promise-against-severe-epilepsy.

Rahn, Bailey. July 21, 2014. "Cannabis and ADD/ADHD." *Leafly*, https://www.leafly.com/news/health/cannabis-and-addadhd/.

Rajesh, Mohanraj, Partha Mukhopadhyay, Sándor Bátkai, Vivek Patel, Keita Saito, Shingo Matsumoto, Yoshihiro Kashiwaya, Béla Horváth, Bani Mukhopadhyay, Lauren Becker, György Haskó, Lucas Liaudet, David A. Wink, Aristidis Veves, Raphael Mechoulam, and Pál Pacher. December 14, 2010. "Cannabidiol attenuates cardiac dysfunction, oxidative stress, fibrosis, and inflammatory and cell death signaling pathways in diabetic cardiomyopathy." *Journal of the American College of Cardiology* 56 (25): 2115–25, doi:10.1016/j.jacc.2010.07.033.

Ramer, Robert, Katharina Bublitz, Nadine Freimuth, Jutta Merkord, Helga Rohde, Maria Haustein, Philipp Borchert, Ellen Schmuhl, Michael Linnebacher, and Burkhard Hinz. April 2012. "Cannabidiol inhibits lung cancer cell invasion and metastasis via intercellular adhesion molecule-1." *FASEB Journal: Official Publication of the Federation of American Societies for Experimental Biology* 26 (4): 1535–48, doi:10.1096/fj.11–198184.

Reichard, Zach. May 16, 2013. "Cannabis: keeping your insulin levels and pant size down." *MedicalJane*, https://www.medicaljane.com/2013/05/16/cannabis-keeping-your-insulin-levels-pant-size-down/.

Rhyne, Danielle N., Sarah L. Anderson, Margaret Gedde, and Laura M. Borgelt. May 2016. "Effects of medical marijuana on migraine headache frequency in an adult population." *Pharmacotherapy* 36 (5): 505–10, doi:10.1002/phar.1673.

Russo, Ethan B. February 2008. "Cannabinoids in the management of difficult to treat pain." *Therapeutics and Clinical Risk Management* 4 (1): 245–59.

Salazar, María, Arkaitz Carracedo, Íñigo J. Salanueva, Sonia Hernández-Tiedra, Mar Lorente, Ainara Egia, Patricia Vázquez, Cristina Blázquez, Sofía Torres, Stephane García, Jonathan Nowak, Gian María Fimia, Mauro Piacentini, Francesco Cecconi, Pier Paolo Pandolfi, Luis González-Feria, Juan L. Iovanna, Manuel Guzmán, Patricia Boya, and Guillermo Velasco. May 1, 2009. "Cannabinoid action induces autophagy-mediated cell death through stimulation of ER stress in human glioma cells." *Journal of Clinical Investigation* 119 (5): 1359–72, doi:10.1172/JCI37948.

Sallan, Stephen E., Norman E. Zinberg, and Emil Frei. October 16, 1975. "Antiemetic effect of delta-9-tetrahydrocannabinol in patients receiving cancer chemotherapy." *New England Journal of Medicine* 293 (16): 795–97, doi:10.1056/NEJM197510162931603.

Sánchez-Duffhues, Gonzalo, Marco A. Calzado, Amaya García de Vinuesa, Francisco J. Caballero, Abdellah Ech-Chahad, Giovanni Appendino, Karsten Krohn, Bernd L. Fiebich, and Eduardo Muñoz. November 15, 2008. "Denbinobin, a naturally occurring 1,4-phenanthrenequinone, inhibits HIV-1 replication through an nf-kappab-dependent pathway." *Biochemical Pharmacology* 76 (10): 1240–50, doi:10.1016/j.bcp.2008.09.006.

Solinas, M., P. Massi, A. R. Cantelmo, M. G. Cattaneo, R. Cammarota, D. Bartolini, V. Cinquina, M. Valenti, L. M. Vicentini, D. M. Noonan, A. Albini, and D. Parolaro. November 2012. "Cannabidiol inhibits angiogenesis by multiple mechanisms." *British Journal of Pharmacology* 167 (6): 1218–31, doi:10.1111/j.1476–5381.2012.02050.x.

Sun Sentinel. August 9, 1990. "Natural 'marijuana' found in brain: Discovery of receptors for cannabis may lead to therapeutic drugs." *Tribunedigital-SunSentinel*, http://articles.sun-sentinel.com/1990-08-09/news/9002080095_1_receptors-cannabinoid-cells.

TruthOnPot.com. November 2, 2012. "Does marijuana cause brain damage?" http://www.truthonpot.com/2012/11/02/does-marijuana-cause-brain-damage/.

Wilkey, Robin. September 19, 2012. "Marijuana and cancer: Scientists find cannabis compound stops metastasis in aggressive cancers." *Huffington Post*, http://www.huffingtonpost.com/2012/09/19/marijuana-and-cancer_n_1898208.html.

CHAPTER 2: WHAT YOGA CAN DO FOR YOU

Alderman, B. L., R. L. Olson, C. J. Brush, and T. J. Shors. February 2, 2016. "MAP training: Combining meditation and aerobic exercise reduces depression and rumination while enhancing synchronized brain activity." *Translational Psychiatry* 6 (2): e726, doi:10.1038/tp.2015.225.

Berrueta, Lisbeth, Igla Muskaj, Sara Olenich, Taylor Butler, Gary J. Badger, Romain A. Colas, Matthew Spite, Charles N. Serhan, and Helene M. Langevin. July 2016. "Stretching impacts inflammation resolution in connective tissue." *Journal of Cellular Physiology* 231 (7): 1621–27, doi:10.1002/jcp.25263.

Boykin, Jade Catherine. 2014. "Physiological and biochemical consequences of sleep deprivation." Biology Honors Program Thesis, Georgia Southern University, http://digitalcommons.georgiasouthern.edu/cgi/viewcontent.cgi?article=1052&context=honors-theses.

Fuss, Johannes, Jörg Steinle, Laura Bindila, Matthias K. Auer, Hartmut Kirchherr, Beat Lutz, and Peter Gass. October 20, 2015. "A runner's high depends on cannabinoid receptors in mice." *Proceedings of the National Academy of Sciences* 112 (42): 13105–8, doi:10.1073/pnas.1514996112.

Harvard Health Publications. March 18, 2016. "Understanding the stress response." http://www.health.harvard.edu/staying-healthy/understanding-the-stress-response.

Johns Hopkins Medicine. Accessed September 11, 2016. "Adrenal glands." http://www.hopkinsmedicine.org/healthlibrary/conditions/endocrinology/adrenal_glands_85,P00399/.

Lamb, Trisha. Accessed September 11, 2016. "Health benefits of yoga." *International Association of Yoga Therapists (IAYT),* http://www.iayt .org/?page=HealthBenefitsOfYoga.

Mayo Clinic. April 21, 2016. "Chronic stress puts your health at risk." http://www.mayoclinic.org/healthy-lifestyle/stress-management/in-depth/stress/art-20046037.

McGreevey, Sue. January 21, 2011. "Eight weeks to a better brain." *Harvard Gazette,* http://news.harvard.edu/gazette/story/2011/01/eight-weeks-to-a-better-brain/.

Möhler, Hanns. January 2012. "The GABA system in anxiety and depression and its therapeutic potential." *Neuropharmacology* 62 (1): 42–53, doi:10.1016/j .neuropharm.2011.08.040.

Streeter, Chris C., J. Eric Jensen, Ruth M. Perlmutter, Howard J. Cabral, Hua Tian, Devin B. Terhune, Domenic A. Ciraulo, and Perry F. Renshaw. May 2007. "Yoga asana sessions increase brain GABA levels: A pilot study." *Journal of Alternative and Complementary Medicine* 13 (4): 419–26, doi:10.1089/acm.2007.6338.

Thirthalli, J., G. H. Naveen, M. G. Rao, S. Varambally, R. Christopher, and B. N. Gangadhar. July 2013. "Cortisol and antidepressant effects of yoga." *Indian Journal of Psychiatry* 55 (Suppl 3): S405–8, doi:10.4103/0019–5545.116315.

University of Mississippi Medical Center. Accessed September 11, 2016. "Physical exercise: Regional blood flow." http://www.umc.edu/Education/ Schools/Medicine/Basic_Science/Physiology_and_Biophysics/Core_ Facilities(Physiology)/Physical_Exercise_-_Regional_Blood_Flow.aspx.

CHAPTER 3: YOGA AND CANNABIS

Kumar, V. Krishna. April 20, 2012. "Cannabis and creativity." *Psychology Today* (blog), http://www.psychologytoday.com/blog/psychology-masala/201204/ cannabis-and-creativity.

National Institute on Alcohol Abuse and Alcoholism. April 1996. "Alcohol and stress." *National Institute on Alcohol Abuse and Alcoholism,* no. 32, PH 363, http://pubs.niaaa.nih.gov/publications/aa32.htm.

CHAPTER 4: THE HISTORY OF CANNABIS AND YOGA

Anday, Jenine K., and Richard W. Mercier. December 2005. "Gene ancestry of the cannabinoid receptor family." *Pharmacological Research* 52 (6): 463–66, doi:10.1016/j.phrs.2005.07.005.

Anthony, David. 2007. *The Horse, the Wheel, and Language: How Bronze-Aged Riders from the Eurasian Steppes Shaped the Modern World.* Princeton, NJ: Princeton Univ. Press, 362.

Bennett, Chris. 2010. *Cannabis and the Soma Solution.* Walterville, OR: Trine Day, 476–82.

Biser, Jennifer A. 1998. "Really wild remedies: Medicinal plant use by animals." *ZooGoer* 27/1, http://westerlymsscience.pbworks.com/f/Really%20Wild%20

Remedies-Medicinal%20Plant%20Use%20by%20Animals%20-%20
National%20Zoo%20FONZ.pdf.

Blaszczak-Boxe, Agata. December 10, 2014. "Drugs in early Americas included
'magic' mushrooms and toad skins." *Live Science,* http://www.livescience
.com/49074-hallocinogens-drugs-early-mesoamerica.html.

Bloomfield, Maurice. Accessed September 16, 2016. *Hymns of the Atharva Veda,*
http://www.sacred-texts.com/hin/av.htm.

Buhler, George, trans. Accessed September 12, 2016. "Laws of Manu." *Sacred
Books of the East, vol. 25,* http://www.sacred-texts.com/hin/manu.htm.

Clark, Walter Houston. Accessed September 12, 2016. "Drug Cult." *Encyclopedia
Britannica,* https://www.britannica.com/topic/drug-cult.

Clarke, Robert, and Mark Merlin. 2013. *Cannabis: Evolution and Ethnobotany.*
Berkeley, CA: Univ. of California Press, 44, 102.

Curry, Andrew. Accessed November 17, 2016. "Gold artifacts tell tale of drug-
fueled rituals and 'bastard wars.'" *National Geographic* online.

Grierson, G. A. 1893–94. "On references to the hemp plant occurring in Sanskrit
and Hindi literature." *Indian Hemp Drugs Commission Report* (Simla, India)
3: 247–48.

Griffin, Ralph T. H., trans. 1896. *Rig Veda,* bk. 8, hymn 68, l. 3, http://www
.sacred-texts.com/hin/rigveda/rv08048.htm.

Gross, Terry. June 1, 2015. "Those yoga poses may not be ancient after all, and
maybe that's OK." *National Public Radio,* http://www.npr.org/sections/
health-shots/2015/06/01/411202468/those-yoga-poses-may-not-be-ancient-
after-all-and-maybe-thats-ok.

Guerra-Doce, Elisa. January 2, 2015. "Psychoactive substances in prehistoric
times: examining the archaeological evidence." *Time and Mind* 8 (1):
91–112, doi:10.1080/1751696X.2014.993244.

Gumbiner, Jann. May 10, 2011. "History of cannabis in ancient China."
   Psychology Today (blog), http://www.psychologytoday.com/blog/the-
   teenage-mind/201105/history-cannabis-in-ancient-china.

————. June 16, 2011. "History of cannabis in India." *Psychology Today* (blog),
   http://www.psychologytoday.com/blog/the-teenage-mind/201106/history-
   cannabis-in-india.

Haynes, Andrew. December 17, 2010. "The animal world has its junkies too."
   Pharmaceutical Journal 285: 783, http://www.pharmaceutical-journal.com/
   opinion/comment/the-animal-world-has-its-junkies-too/11052360.article.

Herodotus. *The Persian Wars,* 4:73–75, http://mcadams.posc.mu.edu/txt/ah/
   Herodotus/Herodotus4.html.

Leafly. Accessed August, 2016. www.leafly.com/news/cannabis-101/cannabis-
   evolution-what-do-we-know-about-the-plants-earliest-orig.

Long, Tengwen, Mayke Wagner, Dieter Demske, Christian Leipe, and Pavel E.
   Tarasov. June 27, 2016. "Cannabis in Eurasia: Origin of human use and
   Bronze Age trans-continental connections." *Vegetation History and
   Archaeobotany,* doi:10.1007/s00334–016–0579–6.

Mathre, Mary Lynn, ed. 1997. *Cannabis in Medical Practice: A Legal, Historical
   and Pharmacological Overview of the Therapeutic Use of Marijuana.*
   Jefferson, NC: McFarland, 35.

Merlin, M. D. 2003. "Archaeological evidence for the tradition of psychoactive
   plant use in the old world." *Economic Botany* 57 (3): 295–323 (301–2, 312),
   http://www.botany.hawaii.edu/plant/wp-content/uploads/2014/04/Merlin-
   2003-article-in-Economic-Botany.pdf.

Sulak, Dustin. Accessed August 2016. "Introduction to the endocannabinoid
   system." *NORML,* http://norml.org/library/item/introduction-to-the-
   endocannabinoid-system.

CHAPTER 6: MEDICATED MINDFULNESS

Åkerstedt, Torbjörn. 2006. "Psychosocial stress and impaired sleep." *Scandinavian Journal of Work, Environment & Health* 32 (6): 493–501.

American Psychology Association. February 23, 2006. "Stress weakens the immune system." http://www.apa.org/research/action/immune.aspx.

Boykin, Jade Catherine. 2014. "Physiological and biochemical consequences of sleep deprivation." Biology honors program thesis, Georgia Southern University, http://digitalcommons.georgiasouthern.edu/cgi/viewcontent. cgi?article=1052&context=honors-theses.

Gopnik, Adam. May 16, 2016. "Feel Me." *New Yorker,* http://www.newyorker. com/magazine/2016/05/16/what-the-science-of-touch-says-about-us.

Kowalski, Kathleen M., and Charles Vaught. Accessed September 14, 2016. "Judgment and decision-making under stress: An overview for emergency managers." *Centers for Disease Control and Prevention,* http://www.cdc.gov/ niosh/mining/UserFiles/works/pdfs/jadmus.pdf.

Mitchell, Marilyn. March 29, 2013. "Dr. Herbert Benson's relaxation response." *Psychology Today* (blog), http://www.psychologytoday.com/blog/heart-and-soul-healing/201303/dr-herbert-benson-s-relaxation-response.

Moseley, G. Lorimer. Accessed September 14, 2016. "Reconceptualising pain according to modern pain science." *Body in Mind,* http://www.bodyinmind. org/resources/journal-articles/full-text-articles/reconceptualising-pain-according-to-modern-pain-science/.

Russ, Tom C., Emmanuel Stamatakis, Mark Hamer, John M. Starr, Mika Kivimäki, and G. David Batty. July 31, 2012. "Association between psychological distress and mortality: Individual participant pooled analysis of 10 prospective cohort studies." *British Medical Journal* 345: e4933, doi:10.1136/bmj.e4933.

Sulak, Dustin. Accessed August 2016. "Introduction to the endocannabinoid system." *NORML,* http://norml.org/library/item/introduction-to-the-endocannabinoid-system.

CHAPTER 7: SAFE STONERS

Krucoff, Carol. August 28, 2007. "Insight from injury." *Yoga Journal,* http://www.yogajournal.com/article/lifestyle/insight-from-injury/.

CHAPTER 8: INTENTION SETTING

West, Jane, and Kristen Williams. January 1, 2016. *Coming Clean with Cannabis: A New Kind of Cleanse.* https://cdn.shopify.com/s/files/1/1000/0656/files/CannabisCleanse-Desktop.pdf?123202971987254742671.

CHAPTER 9: HOW TO ENHANCE

Boyles, Salynn. May 23, 2006. "Pot smoking not linked to lung cancer." *WebMD,* http://www.webmd.com/lung-cancer/news/20060523/pot-smoking-not-linked-to-lung-cancer.

Burstein, S., and S. Hunter. 1995. "Stimulation of anandamide biosynthesis in N-18TG2 neuroblastoma cells by δ^9-tetrahydrocannabinol (THC)." *Biochemical Pharmacology* 49 (6): 855–58.

Crowell, P. L., and M. N. Gould. 1994. "Chemoprevention and therapy of cancer by D-Limonene." *Critical Reviews in Oncogenesis* 5 (1): 1–22.

Dorm, Drake. September 23, 2013. "Terpenes may improve effectiveness of medical cannabis." *MedicalJane,* https://www.medicaljane.com/2013/09/23/terpenes-may-improve-effectiveness-of-medical-marijuana/.

Earlenbaugh, Emily. August 24, 2016. "Are terpene-enriched cannabis concentrates bad for your health?" *Cannabis Now,* https://www.cannabisnow.com/current-events/terpene-cannabis-concentrates-health.

El-Alfy, Abir T., Kelly Ivey, Keisha Robinson, Safwat Ahmed, Mohamed Radwan, Desmond Slade, Ikhlas Khan, Mahmoud ElSohly, and Samir Ross. June 2010. "Antidepressant-like effect of Δ9-tetrahydrocannabinol and other cannabinoids isolated from Cannabis sativa L." *Pharmacology Biochemistry and Behavior* 95 (4): 434–42, doi:10.1016/j.pbb.2010.03.004.

Gieringer, Dale. Summer 1996, updated February 2000. "Marijuana pipe and vaporizer study." *Newsletter for the Multidisciplinary Association of Psychedelic Studies* 6 (3.

Lima, N. G., D. P. De Sousa, F. C. Pimenta, M. F. Alves, F. S. De Souza, R. O. Macedo, R. B. Cardoso, L. C. de Morais, M. D. Melo Diniz, and R. N. de Almeida. September 2012. "Anxiolytic-like activity and GC-MS analysis of (R)-(+)-limonene fragrance, a natural compound found in foods and plants." Pharmacology, Biochemistry and Behavior, Departamento de Ciências Farmacêuticas da Universidade Federal da Paraíba, CEP 58051–970, João Pessoa, Paraíba, Brazil.

Linck, Viviane Moura, Adriana Lourenço da Silva, Micheli Figueiró, Angelo Luis Piato, Ana Paula Herrmann, Franciele Dupont Birck, Elina Bastos Caramão, Domingos Sávio Nunes, Paulo Roberto H. Moreno, and Elaine Elisabetsky. April 2009. "Inhaled linalool-induced sedation in mice." *Phytomedicine: International Journal of Phytotherapy and Phytopharmacology* 16 (4): 303–7, doi:10.1016/j.phymed.2008.08.001.

Ma, Jianqun, Hai Xu, Jun Wu, Changfa Qu, Fenglin Sun, and Shidong Xu. December 2015. "Linalool inhibits cigarette smoke-induced lung inflammation by inhibiting NF-κB activation." *International Immunopharmacology* 29 (2): 708–13, doi:10.1016/j.intimp.2015.09.005.

MedicalJane. Accessed September 14, 2016. "Terpenes: Learn how terpenes work synergistically with cannabinoids." *MedicalJane,* https://www.medicaljane.com/category/cannabis-classroom/terpenes/.

Rahn, Bayley. February 12, 2014. "Terpenes: The flavors of cannabis aromatherapy." *Leafly,* https://www.leafly.com/news/cannabis-101/terpenes-the-flavors-of-cannabis-aromatherapy/.

Rastogi, Nina. March 17, 2009. "Dirty Butts." *Slate,* http://www.slate.com/articles/health_and_science/the_green_lantern/2009/03/dirty_butts.2.html.

Russo, Ethan B. August 2011. "Taming THC: Potential cannabis synergy and phytocannabinoid-terpenoid entourage effects." *British Journal of Pharmacology* 163 (7): 1344–64, doi:10.1111/j.1476–5381.2011.01238.x.

Sun, Jidong. September 2007. "D-limonene: Safety and clinical applications." *Alternative Medicine Review: A Journal of Clinical Therapeutic* 12 (3): 259–64.

Wilsey, Barth, Thomas D. Marcotte, Reena Deutsch, Ben Gouaux, Staci Sakai, and Haylee Donaghe. February 2013. "Low-dose vaporized cannabis significantly improves neuropathic pain." *Journal of Pain* 14 (2): 136–48, doi:10.1016/j.jpain.2012.10.009.

CHAPTER 10: PURCHASING TIPS

Bruso, Jessica. July 8, 2015. "Do hemp seeds contain healthy omega-3 fatty acids?" *Livestrong,* http://www.livestrong.com/article/478632-do-hemp-seeds-contain-healthy-omega-3-fatty-acids/.

Clarke, Thomas H. October 15, 2014. "Hemp oil hustlers: Project CBD investigates makers of RSHO." *Daily Chronic,* http://www.thedailychronic.net/2014/37614/hemp-oil-hustlers-project-cbd-investigates-makers-of-rsho/2/.

Dorm, Drake. August 19, 2013. "Cannabinol (CBN): The cannabinoid that helps you sleep." *MedicalJane,* https://www.medicaljane.com/2013/08/19/cannabinol-cbn-will-put-you-to-bed/.

———. August 3, 2013. "An overview of the cannabinoid cannabigerol (CBG)." *MedicalJane,* https://www.medicaljane.com/2013/08/03/cannabigerol-cbg-is-a-minor-cannabinoid-with-major-impact/.

DrugScience.org. Accessed November 17, 2016. "The 2002 Petition to Reschedule Cannabis." http://www.drugscience.org/dl/dl_comparison.html.

Kannell, Erica. Accessed September 15, 2016. "Benefits of organic hemp protein powder." *HealthyEating,* http://healthyeating.sfgate.com/benefits-organic-hemp-protein-powder-8778.html.

Leaf Science. September 21, 2013. "5 health benefits of cannabichromene (CBC)." *LeafScience,* http://www.leafscience.com/2013/09/21/5-health-benefits-of-cannabichromene-cbc/.

Longo, Marie C., Christine E. Hunter, Robert J. Lokan, Jason M. White, and Michael A. White. 2000. "The prevalence of alcohol, cannabinoids, benzodiazepines, and stimulants amongst injured drivers and their role in driver culpability, part II: The relationship between drug prevalence and drug concentration and driver culpability." *Accident Analysis and Prevention* 32: 623–32.

Migoya, David. September 7, 2015. "Months after marijuana holds, post tests find pesticides in products." *Denver Post,* http://www.denverpost.com/2015/09/07/months-after-marijuana-holds-post-tests-find-pesticides-in-products/.

Mihoc, Marcela, Georgeta Pop, Ersilia Alexa, and Isidora Radulov. October 23, 2012. "Nutritive quality of Romanian hemp varieties (Cannabis sativa L.) with special focus on oil and metal contents of seeds." *Chemistry Central Journal* 6 (1): 122, doi:10.1186/1752–153X-6–122.

Montserrat-de la Paz, S., F. Marín-Aguilar, M. D. García-Giménez, and M. A. Fernández-Arche. February 5, 2014. "Hemp (Cannabis sativa L.) seed oil: Analytical and phytochemical characterization of the unsaponifiable fraction." *Journal of Agricultural and Food Chemistry* 62 (5): 1105–10, doi:10.1021/jf404278q.

Oxenham, Simon. April 20, 2016. "Sativa vs. indica: Fact or fiction?" *PrimeMind,* https://primemind.com/sativa-vs-indica-science-or-folklore-5b6ba6eaaa0d#.t5kbt6cr6.

Piomelli, Daniele. 2016. "The *Cannabis sativa* versus *Cannabis indica* debate: An interview with Ethan Russo, MD," *Cannabis and Cannabinoid Research* 1.1, http://online.liebertpub.com/doi/pdf/10.1089/can.2015.29003.ebr.

Poursafa, Parinaz, Mohammad Mehdi Amin, Parisa Seyed Hoseini, Faramarz Moattar, and Amir Hossein Rezaei. 2012. "Ability of phytoremediation for absorption of strontium and cesium from soils using cannabis sativa." *International Journal of Environmental Health Engineering* 1 (1): 17, doi:10.4103/2277–9183.96004.

Russo, Ethan B. August 2011. "Taming THC: Potential cannabis synergy and phytocannabinoid-terpenoid entourage effects." *British Journal of Pharmacology* 163 (7): 1344–64, doi:10.1111/j.1476–5381.2011.01238.x.

Smith, Phillip. August 7, 2015. "Blowing up the big myths about Indica v. sativa strains of marijuana." *AlterNet,* http://www.alternet.org/drugs/indicas-sativas-myrcene.

Warf, Barney. October 1, 2014. "High points: An historical geography of cannabis." *Geographical Review* 104 (4): 414–38, doi:10.1111/j.1931–0846.2014.12038.x.

CHAPTER 11: ENHANCING

Rosenthal, Ed. 2001. *The Big Book of Buds: Marijuana Varieties from the World's Great Seed Breeders.* Oakland, CA: Quick American Archives.

CHAPTER 12: BAKED BREATHING PRACTICES.

Hancox, R. J., R. Poulton, M. Ely, D. Welch, D. R. Taylor, C. R. McLachlan, J. M. Greene, T. E. Moffitt, A. Caspi, and M. R. Sears. January 2010. "Effects of cannabis on lung function: A population-based cohort study." *European Respiratory Journal* 35 (1): 42–47, doi:10.1183/09031936.00065009.

Harvard Health Publications. March 18, 2016. "Relaxation Techniques: Breath control helps quell errant stress response." http://www.health.harvard.edu/mind-and-mood/relaxation-techniques-breath-control-helps-quell-errant-stress-response.

Jerath, Ravinder, John W. Edry, Vernon A. Barnes, and Vandna Jerath. 2006. "Physiology of long pranayamic breathing: Neural respiratory elements may provide a mechanism that explains how slow deep breathing shifts the autonomic nervous system." *Medical Hypotheses* 67 (3): 566–71, doi:10.1016/j.mehy.2006.02.042.

Pletcher, Mark J., Eric Vittinghoff, Ravi Kalhan, Joshua Richman, Monika Safford, Steve Sidney, Feng Lin, and Stefan Kertesz. January 11, 2012. "Association between marijuana exposure and pulmonary function over 20 years." *Journal of the American Medical Association* 307 (2): 173–81, doi:10.1001/jama.2011.1961.

CHAPTER 13: POSES FOR POTHEADS, PART I

Appleton, Bradford. October 12, 1994. "Stretching and flexibility," *University of Bath Personal Home Pages,* http://people.bath.ac.uk/masrjb/Stretch/stretching_3.html#SEC27.

Bowman, Katy. February 12, 2012. "Hypermobility." *Nutritious Movement* (blog), https://nutritiousmovement.com/hypermobility/.

———. 2014. *Move Your DNA: Restore Your Health Through Natural Movement.* Carlsborg, WA: Propriometrics Press, 124.

Hamblin, James. August 24, 2016. "Why one neuroscientist started blasting his core." *Atlantic,* http://www.theatlantic.com/science/archive/2016/08/cortical-adrenal-orchestra/496679/.

Mense, Siegfried, David Simons, and I. Jon Russell. 2001. *Muscle Pain: Understanding Its Nature, Diagnosis, and Treatment.* Philadelphia: Lippincott, Williams & Wilkins, 265.

Willette, Allen. December 9, 2010. "How muscles heal." *Body in Balance,* http://bodyinbalance.com/856/muscular-injury-pain-muscle-healing/.

CHAPTER 14: POSES FOR POTHEADS, PART 2

Smith, Eva Norlyk. February 5, 2014. "Creating change: Tom Myers on yoga, fascia and mind-body transformation." *Huffington Post,* http://www.huffingtonpost.com/eva-norlyk-smith-phd/mind-body-_b_4387093.html.

CHAPTER 15: MARIJUANA MEDITATIONS

Feldman, Greg, Jeff Greeson, and Joanna Senville. October 2010. "Differential effects of mindful breathing, progressive muscle relaxation, and loving-kindness meditation on decentering and negative reactions to repetitive thoughts." *Behaviour Research and Therapy* 48 (10): 1002–11. http://www.sciencedirect.com/science/article/pii/S0005796710001324.

Fonseca, Fernando Rodríguez de, Ignacio Del Arco, Francisco Javier Bermudez-Silva, Ainhoa Bilbao, Andrea Cippitelli, and Miguel Navarro. January 1, 2005. "The endocannabinoid system: Physiology and pharmacology." *Alcohol and Alcoholism* 4 (1): 2–14, doi:10.1093/alcalc/agh110.

Singh, Yogesh, Ratna Sharma, and Anjana Talwar. November/December 2012. "Immediate and long-term effects of meditation on acute stress reactivity, cognitive functions, and intelligence." *Alternative Therapies in Health and Medicine* 18 (6): 46–53. http://search.proquest.com/openview/4ebae4ab530e7 3e7259475773c6d7c75/1?pq-origsite=gscholar.

Sun Sentinel. August 9, 1990. "Natural 'marijuana' found in brain: Discovery of receptors for cannabis may lead to therapeutic drugs." Tribunedigital-Sunsentinel, 2016. http://articles.sun-sentinel.com/1990-08-09/ news/9002080095_1_receptors-cannabinoid-cells.

INDEX

Page numbers in *italics* refer to illustrations.

enlightenment (*continued*)
210; definition of, 36–37
entheogens, 34
entourage effect, 10, 118
escapism, 143–44
ethics, 158
Europe, 48, 51
evolution, and cannabis, 47–51

fascia, 11, 167, 170, 194
fasting, 145
feeling, 28–30
feminism, 87
fiber, 120
fibromyalgia, 7
fight or flight response, 17
flexibility, 162, 163, 164, 166, 191; stretching and, 165–73
food, 64, 119, 121, 125, 226–27; cannabis smoothies and milkshakes, 222–25; edibles, 98–99; to enhance endocannabinoid system, 226–27
free radicals, 95
friends, 228; Ganja Yoga at home with, 130–32
fungi, 47, 48

GABA, 14, 91, 119, 144
gamma linolenic acid, 120
Ganja Milkshake, Ancient, 224–25
Ganja Yoga, 23–39, 123–47, 218–21; altered states and, 31–39, 83, 123; anxiety and, 136–38; benefits of, 26–35, 220–21; breathing and, 153–55; cannabis dependency and, 143–46, 233–34; cannabis-enhanced yoga class, 127–28, 131; clumsiness and, 142–43; creativity

and, 31; critiques of, 230–35; distraction and, 141–42; doing it alone, 132–33; embodiment and, 28–30; history of, 41–51; at home with friends, 130–32; how to enhance, 89–109; intention setting and, 83–87; lethargy and, 138–40; meditation and, 199–217; mindset, 125–26; practice of poses, 179–97; purchasing tips, 111–21; regular yoga class while high, 128–30, 131; relaxation and, 26–27; ritual, 85–87; safety, 73, 80–81; setting, 124; sex and, 30–31; spirituality and, 23–39, 231; stretching, 165–73; theory of poses, 157–77; troubleshooting, 135–46; when to get high, 133–35; where to do, 126–33
gastrointestinal diseases, 7, 17
glaucoma, 3, 119
glycerin tincture, 100
goals, 87
Goddess worship, 87
Gonur, 51
Google, 60
Green Smoothie, New, 222–23
grinder tips, 97
Gupta, Sanjay, 220
guru (term), 51
GW Pharmaceuticals, 10
gymnastics, 42

Hatha Yoga, 130, 163
heart disease, 7, 8, 17, 25, 65
heart rate, 14, 151
heavy metals, 114–15, 118, 121
hemp, 8, 48, 49, 94, 95, 118, 120–21
hemp seeds, 120–21
hemp wick, 94

ABOUT
THE AUTHOR

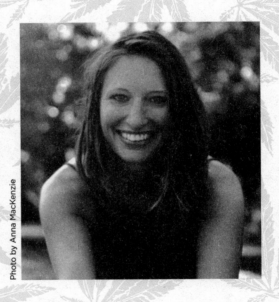

Photo by Anna MacKenzie

DEE DUSSAULT is a 500-hour Yoga Alliance–certified yoga instructor and the first yoga teacher in North America to offer cannabis-enhanced yoga. She holds a degree in sexuality studies from York University. Dee lives in the Bay Area.

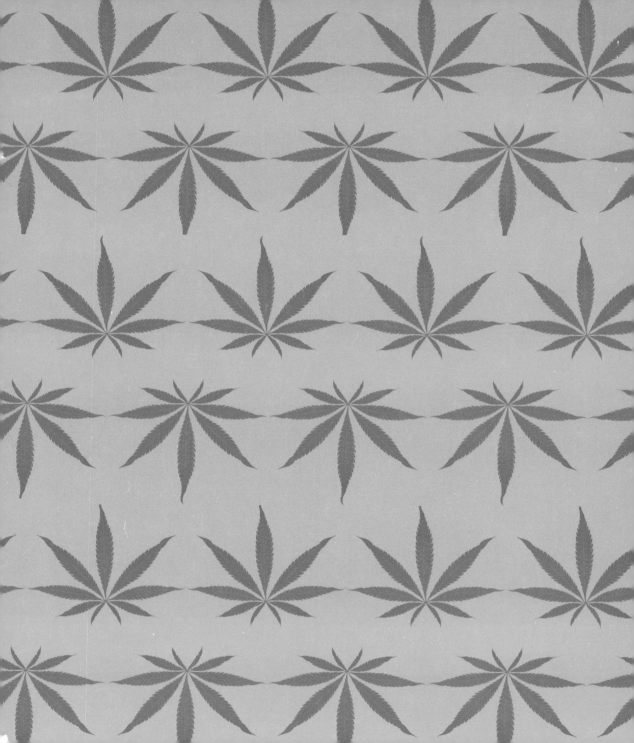